Residues of some veterinary drugs in animals and foods

Monographs prepared by the
Fortieth Meeting of the Joint FAO/WHO
Expert Committee on Food Additives

Geneva, 9-18 June 1992

FAO
FOOD AND
NUTRITION
PAPER
41/5

FOOD
AND
AGRICULTURE
ORGANIZATION
OF THE
UNITED NATIONS
Rome, 1993

The designations employed and the presentation of material in this publication do not imply the expression of any opinion whatsoever on the part of the Food and Agriculture Organization of the United Nations concerning the legal status of any country, territory, city or area or of its authorities, or concerning the delimitation of its frontiers or boundaries.

M-84
ISBN 92-5-103288-2

TABLE OF CONTENTS

	Page
List of Participants	iii
Abbreviations	vii
Introduction	xi
Monographs:	
Closantel	1
Flubendazole	21
Ivermectin	37
Thiabendazole	41
Triclabendazole	63
Furazolidone	87
Nitrofurazone	105
Bovine Somatotropins	113
Ractopamine	143
Isometamedium	155
Annexes:	
1. Summary of JECFA evaluations of veterinary drug residues from the 32nd meeting to the present	167
2. Recommendations on the compounds	173
3. Corrigenda to FAO Food and Nutrition Paper 41/3	177

JOINT FAO/WHO EXPERT COMMITTEE ON FOOD ADDITIVES

Geneva, 9 - 18 June 1992

List of participants

Members invited by FAO

Dr. F.A. Abiola, Chief, Department of Pharmacy and Toxicology of the Inter-State School of Sciences and Veterinary Medecine, Dakar, Senegal

Dr. J. Boisseau, Director, Laboratory of Veterinary Drugs, National Centre of Veterinary and Food Studies, Fougères, France (Vice-Chairman)

Dr. R. Ellis, Director, Chemistry Division, Food Safety and Inspection Service, Department of Agriculture, Washington D.C., USA (Joint Rapporteur)

Dr. P.K. Gupta, Professor and Principal Scientist, Division of Pharmacology and Toxicology, Indian Veterinary Research Institute, Izatnagar, India

Dr. J.L. Rojas Martinez, Chief, Toxicology Section, National Centre for Diagnosis and Research in Animal Health, San José, Costa Rica

Members invited by WHO

Dr. L.-E. Appelgren, Department of Pharmacology and Toxicology, Faculty of Veterinary Medicine, The Swedish University of Agricultural Sciences, Biomedical Centre, Uppsala, Sweden

Dr. D. Arnold, Director, Centre for Surveillance and Health Evaluation of Environmental Chemicals, Berlin, Germany (Joint Rapporteur)

Dr. R.D. Furrow, Deputy Director, Office of New Animal Drug Evaluation, Centre for Veterinary Medicine, Food and Drug Administration, Rockville, MD, USA

Prof. J.G. McLean, Dean, Faculty of Applied Science, Swinburne University of Technology, Hawthorn, Victoria, Australia (Chairman)

Dr. D.M. Pugh, Department of Small Animal Clinical Studies, Faculty of Veterinary Medicine, University College, Dublin, Ireland

Prof. A. Rico, Physiopathology and Experimental Toxicology Laboratory (INRA), Toulouse, France

Secretariat

Mr. D. Byron, Food Quality and Standards Service, Food Policy and Nutrition Division, FAO, Rome, Italy

Dr. R. Fuchs, Head, Department of Toxicology, Institute for Medical Research and Occupational Health, University of Zagreb, Zagreb, Croatia (WHO Temporary Adviser)

Dr. G.B. Guest, Chairman, Codex Committee on Residues of Veterinary Drugs in Foods, Director, Center for Veterinary Medicine, Food and Drug Administration, Rockville, MD, USA

Dr. G. Guyer, Office of New Animal Drug Evaluation, Center for Veterinary Medicine, Food and Drug Administration, Rockville, MD, USA (FAO Consultant)

Dr. R.J. Heitzman, Science Consultant, Newbury, UK (FAO Consultant)

Dr. J.L. Herrman, International Programme on Chemical Safety, WHO, Geneva, Switzerland (Joint Secretary)

Dr. J. Juskevich, Halifax, Nova Scotia, Canada (WHO Temporary Advisor)

Dr. R.C. Livingston, Office of New Animal Drug Evaluation, Center for Veterinary Medicine, Food and Drug Administration, Rockville, MD, USA (FAO Consultant)

Dr. R. Maronpot, Chief, Experimental Toxicology Branch, Division of Toxicology Research and Testing, National Institute of Environmental Health Sciences, Research Triangle Park, NC, USA (WHO Temporary Advisor)

Dr. M. Miller, Antimicrobial and Antiparasitic Drugs Branch, Division of Toxicology and Environmental Sciences, Office of New Animal Drug Evaluation, Center for Veterinary Medicine, Rockville, MD, USA (WHO Temporary Advisor)

Dr. K. Mitsumori, Chief, Third Section, Division of Pathology, Biological Safety Research Center, National Institute of Hygienic Sciences, Tokyo, Japan (WHO Temporary Advisor)

Dr. J. Paakkanen, Ministry of Trade and Industry, Division for Food Affairs, Helsinki, Finland (FAO Consultant)

Dr. L. Ritter, Director, Bureau of Veterinary Drugs, Health Protection Branch, Health and Welfare Canada, Ottawa, Ontario, Canada (WHO Temporary Advisor)

Dr. G. Roberts, Chief Toxicologist, Chemicals Safety Unit, Department of Health, Housing and Community Services, Commonwealth of Australia, Canberra, ACT, Australia (WHO Temporary Advisor)

Dr. F.X.R. van Leeuwen, Toxicology Advisory Centre, National Institute of Public Health and Environmental Protection, Bilthoven, The Netherlands (WHO Temporary Advisor)

Dr. J. Weatherwax, Food Quality and Standards Services, Food Policy and Nutrition Division, FAO, Rome, Italy (Joint Secretary)

Dr. K. Woodward, Veterinary Medicines Directorate, Ministry of Agriculture, Fisheries and Food, Addlestone, Surrey, UK (WHO Temporary Advisor)

ABBREVIATIONS USED IN THIS REPORT

ADI	- Acceptable Daily Intake
a.i.	- Active Ingredient
AUC	- Area Under Curve
BQ	- Below Quantitation Limit
bST	- Bovine SomatoTropin
BW	- Body Weight
°C	- Degrees Celcius
^{14}C	- Radioactive Carbon-14
C18	- Octadecylsilane HPLC reversed phase
c.	- Circa
C_{max}	- Maximum Concentration
cal	- Calorie
μCi	- Microcuries of Radioactivity
cm^3	- Cubic centimeter
conc.	- Concentration
CV	- Coefficient of Variation
DMSO	- DiMethyl SulfOxide
DMF	- DiMethyl Formamide
ECD	- Electron Capture Detection
eq	- Equivalents
F	- Female
°F	- Degrees Fahrenheit
g	- Gram(s)
μg	- Microgram(s)
GC	- Gas Chromatography
GCMS	- Gas Chromatography/Mass Spectrometry
GI	- GastroIntestinal
GLC	- Gas-Liquid Chromatography
h	- Hour(s)
^3H	- Tritium
H_2B_{1a}	- 22,23-Dihydroavermectin-B_{1a}
HPLC	- High Performance Liquid Chromatography
i.e.	- That is
IGF	- Insulin-like Growth Factor
IM	- Intra Muscular
IV	- Intra Venous
kd	- kilodaltons
kg	- Kilogram
L	- Litre
lb(s)	- Pound(s)
LC	- Liquid Chromatography
LWG	- Live Weight Gain
M	- Molar or Mole
MA	- Male
μm	- Micrometre(s)

mg	- Milligram(s)
min	- Minute(s)
ml	- Millilitre(s)
mM	- Millimole(s)
MR	- Marker Residue
MRL	- Maximum Residue Level
MS	- Mass Spectrometry
n	- Number
No	- Number
N	- Normal
^{15}N	- Radioactive Nitrogen-15
NA	- Not Analyzed or Not Assayed
ND	- Not Detected
NDR	- Not Detectable Residue
NEFA	- Nonesterified Fatty Acids
NFA	- 5-Nitro-2-Furaldehyde
ng	- Nanogram(s)
NIH	- National Institute of Health of the United States
nm	- Nanometre(s)
NMR	- Nuclear Magnetic Resonance
NPN	- NonProtein Nitrogen
PAGE	- PolyAcrylamide Gel Electrophoresis
PO	- Per Oral
ppb	- Parts per billion
ppm	- Parts per million
PTH	- ParaThyroid Hormone
q.s.p.	- Quantity sufficient
r	- linearity
rbGH	- Recombinant bovine Growth Hormone
rbST	- Recombinant bovine SomatoTropin
Rec.	- Recommended
RIA	- RadioImmunoAssay
^{35}S	- Radioactive Sulphur-35
SC	- SubCutaneous
SD	- Standard Deviation
SDS	- Sodium Dodecyl Sulfate
SEM	- Standard Error of Mean
SNR	- Signal to Noise Ratio
ST	- SomatoTropin
$t½$	- Half life
t_{max}	- Maximum time
TBZ	- ThiaBendaZole
TLC	- Thin Layer Chromatography
TR	- Total Residue
TRA	- Total RadioActivity
UD	- Unchanged flubendazole
UV	- UltraViolet
v/v	- Volume/volume

w/v	- Weight/volume
WT	- Withdrawal Time
%	- Per cent
~	- Approximately
>	- Greater than
<	- Less than
≤	- Equal or less than

INTRODUCTION

The Monographs on the residues of the ten compounds contained in this volume were prepared by the Fortieth meeting of the Joint FAO/WHO Expert Committee on Food Additives (JECFA), which was held in Geneva, 9 - 18 June 1992. JECFA has evaluated veterinary drugs at previous meetings, including the 12th[1], 26th[2], 27th[3], 32nd[4], 34th[5], 36th[6] and 38th[7] meetings. In response to a growing concern about mass-medication of food producing animals and the implications for human health and international trade, a Joint FAO/WHO Expert Consultation on Residues of Veterinary Drugs was convened in Rome, in November 1984[8]. Among the main recommendations of this consultation were the establishment of a specialized Codex Committee on Residues of Veterinary Drugs in Foods (CCRVDF) and the periodic convening of an appropriate body to provide independent scientific advice to this Committee and to the member countries of FAO and WHO. At its first session in Washington D.C. in November 1986, the newly-created CCRVDF reaffirmed the need for such a scientific body and made a number of recommendations and suggestions to be considered by JECFA[9]. In response to these recommendations , the Thirty-Second JECFA meeting was entirely devoted to the evaluation of residues of veterinary drugs in foods. Subsequently, the 34th, 36th, 38th and 40th meetings of JECFA were also devoted only to evaluation of veterinary drugs.

The fifth session of the CCRVDF, held in Washington D.C. during October 1990, revised the priority list of veterinary drugs requiring evaluation. The drugs evaluated during the 40th meeting of JECFA included these compounds, except rafoxamide which was scheduled by the sixth session of CCRVDF in October 1991 to be evaluated by the 42nd meeting of JECFA. In addition the 40th Meeting of JECFA re-evaluated ivermectin and evaluated isometamedium which was and was to be evaluated by the 36th and 42nd JECFA meeting, respectively.

The present volume contains summary monographs of the residue data on all ten compounds on the agenda. From the five anthelmintics closantel was considered for cattle and sheep, flubendazole for pigs and poultry, ivermectin for cattle, thiabendazole for cattle, pigs, goats and sheep and triclabendazole for cattle and sheep. Closantel and ivermectin had been previously evaluated by the 36th meeting of JECFA. Flubendazole, thiabendazole and triclabendazole had not been previously reviewed by the Expert Committee.

The two antimicrobial agents, furazolidone and nitrofurazone, had not been previously evaluated by the Committee. They were considered in the current evaluation for pigs and chickens.

The two production aids, ractopamine and bovine somatotropins (bST) had not been previously reviewed by the Committee. Ractopamine was considered for pigs and bST for lactating cows.

Trypanocide, isometamedium, previously evaluated at the 34th meeting of the Committee, was considered for cattle only.

The pertinent information in each monograph was discussed and appraised by the entire Committee. The monographs are presented in a uniform format covering identity, residues in food and their evaluation, metabolism studies, methods of residue analysis and a final appraisal of the study results. More recent publications and documents are referenced, including those on which the monograph is based. A summary of the JECFA evaluations from the 32nd to the present 40th meeting is included in Annex 1.

A corrigendum, related to the Benzyl penicillin evaluation published in the FAO Food and Nutrition Paper 41/3, has been appended to this volume as Annex 3.

The assistance of Dr. R. Livingston and Dr. G. Guyer, both of the United States Food and Drug Administration, and of Dr. R. Heitzman, a private consultant, in preparing these monographs is gratefully acknowledged.

REFERENCES

1. Specifications for the Identity and Purity of Food Additives and their Toxicological Evaluation: Some antibiotics (Twelfth Report of the Joint FAO/WHO Expert Committee on Food Additives), FAO Nutrition Meetings Report Series No. 45, 1969; WHO Technical Report Series No. 430, 1969.

2. Evaluation of Certain Food Additives and Contaminants (Twenty-Six Report of the Joint FAO/WHO Expert Committee on Food Additives). WHO Technical Report Series No. 683; 1982.

3. Evaluation of Certain Food Additives and Contaminants (Twenty-Seventh Report of the Joint FAO/WHO Expert Committee on Food Additives). WHO Technical Report Series No. 696; 1983.

4. Evaluation of Certain Veterinary Drug Residues in Foods. (Thirty-Second Report of the Joint FAO/WHO Expert Committee on Food Additives). WHO Technical Report Series No. 763; 1988.

5. Evaluation of Certain Veterinary Drug Residues in Foods. (Thirty-Fourth Report of the Joint FAO/WHO Expert Committee on Food Additives). WHO Technical Report Series No. 788; 1989.

6. Evaluation of Certain Veterinary Drug Residues in Foods. (Thirty-Sixth Report of the Joint FAO/WHO Expert Committee on Food Additives). WHO Technical Report Series No. 799; 1990.

7. Evaluation of Certain Veterinary Drug Residues in Foods. (Thirty-Eighth Report of the Joint FAO/WHO Expert Committee on Food Additives). WHO Technical Report Series No. 815; 1991.

8. Residues of Veterinary Drugs in Foods, Report of a Joint FAO/WHO Consultation, Rome, 29 October - 5 November 1984. FAO Food and Nutrition Paper No. 32, 1985.

9. Report of the First Session of the Codex Committee on Residues of Veterinary Drugs in Foods. Washington D.C., 27-31 October 1986.

CLOSANTEL

IDENTITY

Chemical names: N-[5-chloro-4-[(4-chlorophenyl)cyanomethyl]-2-methylphenyl]-2-hydroxy-3,5-diiodobenzamide

Synonyms: Flukiver
Seponver

Structural formula:

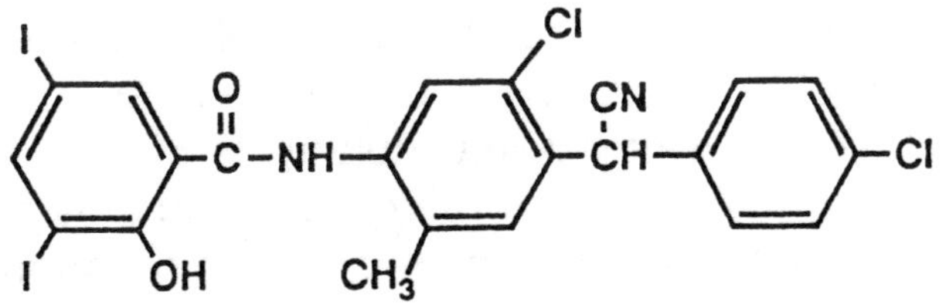

Molecular formula: $C_{22}H_{14}Cl_2I_2N_2O_2$

Molecular weight: 663.08

OTHER INFORMATION ON IDENTITY AND PROPERTIES

Pure active ingredient:

Appearance: Almost white to beige powder

Melting point: 215-235°C with decomposition

RESIDUES IN FOOD AND THEIR EVALUATION

CONDITIONS OF USE

General

Closantel is used primarily in cattle and sheep for the treatment and control of adult and immature liver flukes, haematophagous nematodes and larval stages of some arthropods.

Dosages

Closantel may be administered to sheep and cattle orally or parenterally via drench, bolus or injectable formulations. The common use of the injectable formulation, delivered subcutaneously or intramuscularly, is 5.0 mg/kg in sheep and 2.5 mg/kg in cattle. The dose range for the oral route is primarily 5 to 10 mg/kg in sheep and cattle; however, the use of 15 mg/kg is recommended for treatment of *Fascioloides*, which is a minor indication. A single application of the drug is recommended.

METABOLISM

Pharmacokinetics

The pharmacokinetic studies on absorption, distribution, metabolism, excretion, and tissue depletion that are summarized were conducted using closantel labelled with carbon-14 in the carbonyl carbon of the benzamide ring.

Rat

Five male Wistar rats were given a single oral dose of closantel at 20 mg/kg, provided as a 0.5% suspension. Maximum concentrations of closantel in serum (C_{max}) of 73.1 ± 10.3 μg/ml (X ± 1 SD) occurred at 1 day after administration (t_{max}). Closantel depletion in serum from t_{max} was monoexponential with a $t_{1/2}$ of 2.8 days. The area under the curve ($AUC_{0-\infty}$) was 408 μg·day/ml. (Van Beijsterveldt et al., 1989)

Sheep

Several pharmacokinetic studies have been conducted in sheep but only one with ^{14}C-labelled closantel and it will be summarized.

^{14}C-labelled closantel was administered orally or intramuscularly to two groups of five sheep at doses of 10 and 5 mg/kg, respectively. Peak radioactive plasma concentrations, occurring at 8-24 hours after drug administration, were similar by both routes, amounting to 47.0 ± 11.1 and 47.9 ± 4.4 μg-eq/ml for the oral and intramuscular route respectively. Plasma radioactivity was 86 to 91% unmetabolized drug. Closantel was eliminated from plasma with a $t_{1/2}$ of 26.7 and 22.7 days after oral and intramuscular administration respectively. The $AUC_{0-\infty}$ values for the respective routes were similar, 1303 and 1027 μg·day/ml, indicating that the systemic bioavailability of orally administered closantel is half that of an intramuscular dose.

Within 8 weeks after oral or intramuscular dosing, about 80 % of the administered dose was excreted with the feces, and only 0.5 % with the urine. (Meuldermans, W. et al., 1982)

Cattle

As with sheep, several pharmacokinetic studies have been conducted in cattle but only one with ^{14}C-labelled closantel and it will be summarized.

^{14}C-labelled closantel was administered orally to five Friesian heifers and four Friesian steers at a single dose of 10 mg/kg. The average C_{max} values for total radioactivity (TRA) in blood and plasma were 26.8 and 35.7 μg-eq/ml, occurring after 48 hours (t_{max}). The $AUC_{0-\infty}$ for TRA in plasma was 593 μg-eq·day/ml and a half-life of 11 days. All TRA in the plasma was unmetabolized drug. Within 42 days, 90 % of the dose was excreted with the feces and less than 0.25% in the urine. (Van Leemput et al., 1991)

Metablolism in Food and Laboratory Animals

Rat

Five male Wistar rats (~242 g) were dosed orally with ^{14}C-closantel at 10 mg/kg. The drug, labeled in the carbonyl carbon, had a radiochemical purity of ~97%. Urine and feces were collected at 24-h periods up to 10 days post dosing. Plasma was collected at sacrifice after the 10-day excreta collection period. Samples were analyzed for total radioactivity by combustion and counting or by direct counting. Unchanged drug and metabolites were determined using HPLC co-chromatography with reference standards.

Radioactivity was found to be excreted primarily through the feces. After 10 days, fecal excretion amounted to 88.4% of the dose. Over that same time period, only 0.4% of the dose was in the urine. Approximately half the dose was excreted within 2 days after dosing.

An examination of the feces for metabolites evidenced unchanged closantel (90% of the radioactivity in the feces at 0-24 hr collection period, 76% at 192-240 h) and monoiodoclosantel (3.4% of the sample radioactivity at the first collection, 19% at the last). The monoiodoclosantel is stated to be predominantly the 3-iodo isomer. Also present in feces were deiodinated closantel (trace amounts) and an unidentified metabolite (~3-6% of the fecal radioactivity).

In the urine, closantel and a metabolite that co-eluted with monoiodosalicylic acid were observed. This latter compound would result from reductive deiodination and amide hydrolysis of closantel. No sulfate or glucuronide conjugates were detected.

Total residues of closantel in plasma amounted to 3.54 ppm 10 days after dosing. Even after that 10-day period, closantel was 93.4% of the total radioactivity. Monoiodoclosantel was 4.7% of the plasma radioactivity.

These data demonstrate the similarity of the metabolism of closantel in rats and sheep. The scheme shown in Figure 1 would, therefore, apply to rats, with the possibility of amide hydrolysis occurring after the initial deiodination step. (Mannens et al., 1989)

Sheep

Following the administration of ^{14}C-closantel to sheep via the intramuscular (5 mg/kg) or oral (10 mg/kg) route, parent closantel was found to be the major constituent of the residue in feces (80-90% of the total residue) and in liver (~60-70% of the total residue). In muscle, kidney and fat, the total residue was very nearly attributable to closantel exclusively.

In feces, two metabolites were identified, by reference to standards, to be 3-monoiodoclosantel and 5-monoiodoclosantel. The 3-monoiodoclosantel isomer was present in a larger amount than the 5-isomer. In feces, no evidence of completely deiodinated closantel was found. In liver, closantel was 61% of the total residue after intramuscular treatment and 71% following oral dosing. Monoiodoclosantel was the main metabolite in liver. The metabolic pathways for closantel in sheep are presented in Figure 1.

Figure 1. **Metabolic Pathways of Closantel in Sheep. The Position of ^{14}C is Indicated by the Asterisk.**

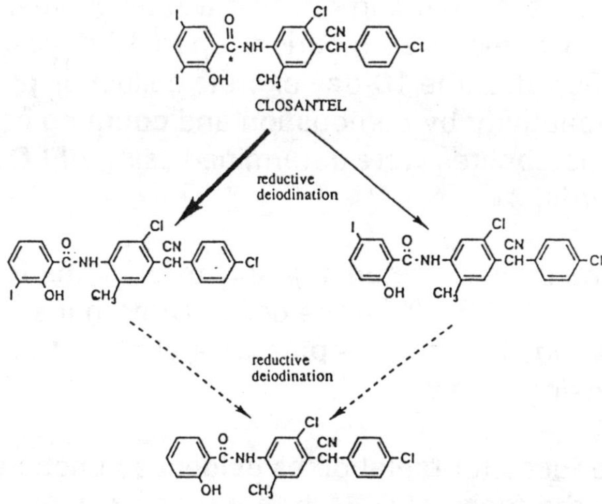

The primary route of metabolism of closantel, therefore, is reductive deiodination leading to the monoiodoclosantel isomers. Although complete deiodination is possible, no evidence for deiodinated closantel has been observed. While amide hydrolysis would appear to be a possible alternate pathway, no metabolites which would result from the pathway (e.g., 3,5-diiodosalicylic acid) have been identified. It may well be that steric hindrance around the amide bonds prevents the hydrolysis. (Meuldermans et al., 1982; Michiels et al., 1987)

Cattle

^{14}C-labelled closantel was administered orally to five Friesian heifers and four Friesian steers at a single dose of 10 mg/kg. Parent closantel was found to be the major constituent in feces (82 % of the total residue) and in kidney, muscle and fat (70-80, 80-100 and 60-100 % of the total residue, respectively). However, unmetabolized closantel only accounted for 6-15 % of the total residue in liver. Characterization of the closantel-derived radioactivity in the liver showed that 40-77 % of the radioactivity could be accounted for by monoiodoclosantel. Further analysis of the monoiodoclosantel revealed that it was the 3-monoiodoclosantel metabolite present, resulting from the deiodination at the 5-position of the benzamide moiety.

Besides the unmetabolized drug, only one notable metabolite was detected in the methanol extracts of the feces. This metabolite accounted for approximately 6% of the administered dose in the feces extracts of the samples collected during the first two weeks. This metabolite also occurred in the bile. Elucidation of this metabolite was performed by mass spectrometry and UV analysis and determined to be a sulfate conjugate of a closantel-derivative where one iodine had been removed and an hydroxyl substituent attached on the benzamide moiety (see Figure 2 below). (Van Leemput et al., 1991)

Figure 2. **Metabolite of Closantel in Cattle Feces and Bile. The Position of ^{14}C is Indicated by the Asterisk.**

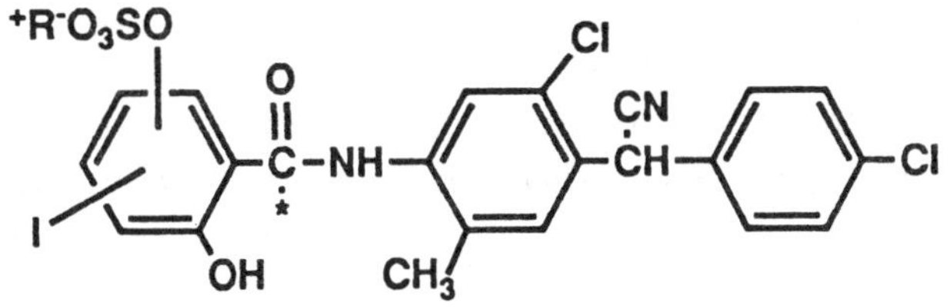

R = H, Na or K

TISSUE RESIDUE DEPLETION STUDIES

Radiolabelled Residue Depletion Studies

Sheep

Five Texel sheep (3MA, 2F) were dosed intramuscularly with 5 mg/kg ^{14}C-closantel while another five (3MA, 2F) were treated orally (stomach tube) with 10 mg/kg labeled drug. The body weights of the sheep ranged from 27 to 35 kg. The ^{14}C-closantel had a specific activity of 23.5 µCi/mg and a radiochemical purity of 97% as determined by radio-HPLC. The labeled drug was diluted with cold drug to give material with a specific activity of 4.2 µCi/mg.

Blood samples were collected on heparin from a jugular vein before and at 4, 8, 24, 48, 96 and 168 hours after drug administration, and weekly up to the time of sacrifice. Urine and feces were collected daily from dosing up to the time of sacrifice. At 14, 21, 35, 42 and 56 days after treatment, one animal from each group was sacrificed. From each animal, samples of liver, muscle, mesenteral fat and kidneys were taken.

Whole blood was analyzed by combustion and liquid scintillation counting, while plasma was measured for radioactivity by direct counting. Urine samples were analyzed by air drying of the sample followed by combustion and counting.

Feces samples were also analyzed by combustion and counting. Tissue samples were homogenized in water and counted directly. The metabolite pattern in some urine, feces, liver or plasma samples was investigated by radio-HPLC.

Peak concentrations of closantel in blood and plasma occurred at 24 h and were similar for both routes of administration (~32 ppm for blood, ~47 ppm for plasma). Closantel was eliminated from plasma with a $t_{1/2}$ of ~27 and ~23 days after oral or intramuscular administration, respectively. By extraction and HPLC analysis of the plasma, it was found that ~90% of the radioactivity represented unchanged closantel.

Analysis of the excreta showed that within 8 weeks after oral or intramuscular dosing ~80% of the administered radioactivity was excreted with the feces and only ~0.5% with the urine. The larger fecal excretion of the radioactivity during the first two days after oral dosing (43.3%) as opposed to intramuscular dosing (10.4%) reflects the smaller systemic availability by the oral route. HPLC analysis of excreta showed that unchanged closantel accounted for 80 to 90% of the eliminated radioactivity. In feces, two other radioactive peaks were detected. These peaks were determined, by reference to standard compounds, to be the 3- and 5-monoiodoclosantel derivatives, indicating reductive deiodination to be a main metabolic pathway. These monoiodoclosantel derivatives were present in urine in only small amounts. Other metabolites in urine, comprising only <0.5% of the total dose, did not correspond to available reference compounds.

The results of assays on tissues for total radioactivity and unchanged closantel are given in Tables 1 and 2 below. Of the edible tissues, kidney contained the highest levels of total residue and closantel. Thus, after intramuscular dosing at 5 mg/kg or oral dosing at 10 mg/kg, kidney contained ~3.3 ppm total residue at 14 days and 1.4 - 1.7 ppm at 56 days ($t_{1/2}$ ~25 days). An examination of the residue in the tissues using HPLC shows that in fat, muscle and kidney virtually all the total residue can be attributed to closantel. In liver, closantel by HPLC represents ~60-70% of the total residue. The main metabolites in liver were shown to be the 3- and 5-monoiodoclosantel derivatives by radio-HPLC. (Meuldermans et al., 1982)

Table 1. Concentration of Total Residue (TR) and Unchanged Closantel (C) in Tissues of Sheep Treated with 5 mg/kg ^{14}C-Closantel Intramuscularly (ppm)

Withdrawal	Muscle		Liver		Kidney		Fat	
Time (days)	TR	C	TR	C	TR	C	TR	C
14	0.59	0.58	2.11	1.59	3.44	3.53	0.25	0.23
21	0.41	0.32	1.95	0.59	2.54	2.45	0.42	0.40
35	0.39	0.35	1.05	0.79	1.83	1.90	0.07	<0.1
42	0.20	0.20	1.00	0.70	1.48	1.42	0.07	<0.1
56	0.19	0.10	0.67	0.36	1.66	1.36	0.09	<0.1

Table 2. Concentration of Total Residue (TR) and Unchanged Closantel (C) in Tissues of Sheep Treated Orally with 10 mg/kg ^{14}C-Closantel (ppm)

Withdrawal	Muscle		Liver		Kidney		Fat	
Time (days)	TR	C	TR	C	TR	C	TR	C
14	0.75	0.78	1.54	1.24	3.27	3.20	0.17	0.17
21	0.75	0.75	1.58	1.15	2.96	2.87	0.08	<0.1
35	0.44	0.39	0.99	0.67	1.97	1.91	0.09	<0.1
42	0.31	0.30	1.92	1.18	2.15	1.95	0.06	<0.1
56	0.24	0.15	0.67	0.49	1.40	0.88	0.11	<0.1

In Table 3, the tissue to plasma ratios for radioactivity are given. It is suggested that the ratios are independent of time and, therefore, that the plasma elimination reflects the depletion of residues from the tissues. (Meuldermans et al., 1982)

Table 3. Tissue to Plasma Ratios of Radioactivity in Sheep After Oral 10 mg/kg (PO) or Intramuscular (IM) 5 mg/kg Dose of ^{14}C-Closantel

Withdrawal	Muscle		Liver		Kidney		Fat	
Time (days)	PO	IM	PO	IM	PO	IM	PO	IM
14	0.039	0.023	0.081	0.083	0.172	0.135	0.009	0.010
21	0.040	0.025	0.084	0.119	0.157	0.155	0.004	0.026
35	0.034	0.033	0.077	0.090	0.153	0.156	0.007	0.006
42	0.016	0.021	0.099	0.107	0.111	0.158	0.003	0.007
56	0.028	0.027	0.078	0.095	0.163	0.235	0.013	0.013
Mean	0.031	0.026	0.084	0.099	0.151	0.168	0.007	0.012

Cattle

Five Friesian heifers and four Friesian steers, weighing 203-252 kg, were administered a single oral dose (via stomach tube) of 10 mg/kg of ^{14}C-labelled closantel. For the 6-week phase, the ^{14}C-closantel had a specific activity of 2.39 μCi/mg and a radiochemical purity of 98.1 % as determined by radio-HPLC. The labeled drug was diluted with cold drug to give material with a specific activity of 1.62 μCi/mg. For the 2- and 4-week phases, the ^{14}C-closantel had a specific activity of 2.12 μCi/mg and a radiochemical purity of 100 % as determined by radio-HPLC. The labeled drug was diluted with cold drug to give material with a specific activity of 2.08 μCi/mg.

For the 6-week phase, there were two heifers and one steer included in the study of the mass balance of the ^{14}C-closantel-derived radioactivity. Blood samples were collected on heparin from a jugular vein before and at 4, 8, 24, 48, 72 and 96 hours after drug administration, and weekly up to 42 days. Urine and feces were collected daily from dosing up to the time of sacrifice. At 42 days after treatment, the three animals were sacrificed. From each animal, samples of liver, muscle, mesenteral fat and kidneys were taken.

For the 2- and 4-week phase, there were three heifers and three steers included in the study of tissue depletion of the ^{14}C-closantel-derived radioactivity. Blood samples were collected on heparin from a jugular vein before and at 4, 8, 24, 48, 72 and 96 hours after drug administration, and weekly up to the time of sacrifice. Urine and feces were collected daily from dosing up to the time of sacrifice. Group 1 was comprised of two heifers and one steer and they were sacrificed at 14 days after treatment. Group 2 was comprised on one heifer and two steers and they were sacrificed at 28 days after treatment. From each animal, samples of liver, muscle, mesenteral fat and kidneys were taken.

Whole blood was analyzed by combustion and liquid scintillation counting, while plasma was measured for radioactivity by direct counting. Urine samples were analyzed by liquid scintillation counting. Feces samples were analyzed by combustion and counting. Tissue samples were homogenized in water and counted directly. The metabolite pattern in some urine, feces, liver or plasma samples was investigated by radio-HPLC.

The results of the pharmacokinetics and metabolism from this study have been described previously in their respective sections.

The results of assays on tissues for total radioactivity and unchanged closantel are given in Table 4. Of the edible tissues, liver contained the highest levels of total residue and kidney contained the highest concentrations of unmetabolized closantel. Thus, after oral dosing at 10 mg/kg, liver contained ~3.7 ppm total residue at 14 days and 1.1 ppm at 42 days. An examination of the residue in the tissues using HPLC shows that in fat, muscle and kidney a large portion of the total residue can be attributed to closantel. Parent closantel accounts for approximately 100, 80 and 70 % of the total residues in muscle, kidney and fat, respectively. In liver, closantel by HPLC represents ~10 % of the total residue. The main metabolite in liver was shown to be the 3-monoiodoclosantel derivative by radio-HPLC. (Van Leemput et al., 1991)

Table 4. Mean Concentration (n=3/group) of Total Residue (TR) and Unchanged Closantel (C) in Tissues of Cattle Treated with 10 mg/kg ^{14}C-Closantel Orally (ppm)

Withdrawal	Muscle		Liver		Kidney		Fat	
Time (days)	TR	C	TR	C	TR	C	TR	C
14	0.71	0.57	3.71	0.54*	2.50	1.87	1.09	0.78
28	0.34	0.37	2.41	0.17*	1.28	1.05	0.83	0.52
42	0.13	0.16*	1.13	≤0.1	0.47	0.38	0.20	0.18

* - This mean does not include one value which was ≤ 0.1 ppm.

In Table 5, the tissue to plasma ratios for radioactivity are given. As with sheep, the data suggest that the ratios are independent of time and, therefore, that the plasma elimination reflects the depletion of residues from the tissues.

Table 5. Tissue to Plasma Ratios of Radioactivity in Cattle After Oral 10 mg/kg (PO) Dose of ^{14}C-Closantel

Withdrawal Time (days)	Muscle	Liver	Kidney	Fat
14	0.044	0.227	0.153	0.067
28	0.044	0.312	0.169	0.108
42	0.050	0.423	0.192	0.077
Mean	0.046	0.321	0.171	0.084

OTHER RESIDUE DEPLETION STUDIES

Sheep

Two groups of 4 sheep (2MA, 2F) weighing 35.7-51.4 kg were treated with closantel either at 5 mg/kg intramuscularly or 10 mg/kg orally. Blood samples were taken from each animal before and at various times after dosing. At 2, 4, 6 and 8 weeks after dosing, one male and one female animal of either group were sacrificed and samples of edible tissues were taken. Samples were analyzed for closantel using a GLC-electron capture method (stated limit of detection, 0.1 ppm) that used an internal standard.

Peak plasma levels of ~50 ppm were reached at 24 h. The drug was eliminated from plasma with a $t_{1/2}$ of ~16 days. The concentrations of closantel in sheep tissues are given in Table 6. Tissue levels were generally comparable for the oral and intramuscular routes. Of the edible tissues, kidney contained the highest concentration of closantel (~2.7 ppm at 14 days). (Michiels et al., 1977a)

Table 6. Concentrations of Closantel (ppm) in Sheep After a Single Oral (PO, 10 mg/kg) or Intramuscular (IM, 5 mg/kg) Dose

Withdrawal	Muscle		Liver		Kidney		Fat	
Time (days)	PO	IM	PO	IM	PO	IM	PO	IM
14	2.0	2.3	1.7	0.9	2.7	2.6	2.6	1.7
28	<0.4	1.1	0.8	0.7	0.7	1.2	0.7	0.4
42	<0.4	<0.5	0.8	0.3	0.6	1.2	0.5	<0.4
56	<0.3	NA	0.4	<0.5	1.2	0.8	0.9	<0.5

Ten sheep (7MA, 3F) weighing 26.9 ± 2.1 kg were treated orally with closantel at 5 mg/kg. Groups of three animals (2MA, 1F) were sacrificed at 14, 18 and 42 days and samples of edible tissues were collected for analysis. A serum sample was taken from the tenth animal at day 56. Closantel was determined with an

HPLC method (limit of detection, 0.1 ppm).

The results of this study are given in Table 7. Levels of closantel at 14 days were highest in kidney (2.43 ppm) and fat (2.17 ppm). By day 42, concentrations of closantel in kidney dropped to 0.62 ppm and in fat to 0.80 ppm. The concentration of closantel in serum was 1.6 ppm. (Michiels et al., 1979)

Table 7. Concentration of Closantel in Tissues of Sheep Treated with a Single Oral Dose of 5 mg/kg (ppm)

Withdrawal Time (days)	Muscle	Liver	Kidney	Fat
14	1.13±0.11	1.00±0.50	2.43±0.71	2.17±0.75
28	0.20±0.07	0.48±0.33	0.78±0.62	0.45±0.26
42	0.22±0.04	0.23±0.09	0.62±0.35	0.80±0.33

Two groups of six sheep weighing 47 ± 11 kg were treated orally with 5 or 10 mg/kg closantel. Three animals of either group were sacrificed 56 days after treatment and the remaining ones after an 84-day withdrawal period. Samples of liver, kidney, muscle and fat were taken for analysis of closantel. Blood samples were collected from all animals every two weeks up to the time of sacrifice. Closantel was measured with an HPLC procedure, limit of detection 0.1 ppm.

In this study, maximal concentrations of closantel in plasma of sheep were 14.5 ppm and 33.9 ppm for the 5 and 10 mg/kg doses at 14 days. The levels for the respective doses decreased with a half-life of ~24 days to 1.7 ppm and 3.8 ppm after 84 days of withdrawal. Residues of closantel in tissues are summarized in Table 8. After the 5 mg/kg dose, residue levels at 56 days were 0.06-0.09 ppm for fat and muscle and up to 0.47 ppm for kidney and liver. At 84 days, residues were not detected in fat and muscle, while they had decreased to 0.06-0.17 ppm for liver and kidney. After the 10 mg/kg dose, residue levels at 56 days were 0.65-0.81 ppm for kidney and liver and 0.19-0.24 ppm for fat and muscle. At 84 days, the residue levels were ~0.1 ppm for liver, fat and muscle and 0.25 ppm for kidney. (Michiels et al., 1980a)

Table 8. Concentration of Closantel in Tissues of Sheep After a Single Oral Dose at 5 or 10 mg/kg (ppm)

Withdrawal	Muscle		Liver		Kidney		Fat	
Time (days)	5	10	5	10	5	10	5	10
14	2.0	2.3	1.7	0.9	2.7	2.6	2.6	1.7
56	0.09	0.24	0.43	0.81	0.47	0.65	0.06	0.19
84	ND	0.13	0.06	0.10	0.17	0.25	ND	0.10

Cattle

Twelve Friesian cattle (6MA, 6F), mean body weight 270 ± 28 kg, were administered a single oral dose of closantel at 10 mg/kg using a 5% suspension formulation (Seponver®). A group of four animals were sacrificed at 14, 28 and 42 days after treatment. Samples of liver, kidney, muscle and fat were taken for analysis of closantel using the validated HPLC method having a detection limit of 0.1 ppm (Woestenborghs et al., 1979; Woestenborghs et al., 1985). Blood samples were collected from all animals before dosing and at 1, 2, 3, 4, 7 and 14 days after administration and from all animals at 21, 28, 35 and 42 days after administration for those animals remaining in the experiment.

The maximum concentrations of closantel in plasma occurred at ~2 days after treatment and were 30.7 µg/ml on average. The $AUC_{0-\infty}$ averaged 517 µg·day/ml and the mean $t_{1/2}$ for the elimination of closantel from plasma was ~11 days.

The highest concentrations of closantel in tissues were found in kidney: from 3.29 ppm at day 14 to 0.11 ppm at day 42. Muscle concentrations ranged from 0.58 ppm at day 14 to ≤ 0.10 ppm at day 42. Concentrations in fat varied from 0.93 ppm to ≤ 0.10 ppm at day 42. Liver concentrations decreased from a maximum of 1.55 ppm after 14 days to ≤ 0.10 ppm at day 42. The mean results are described in Table 9 below. (Van Beijsterveldt et al., 1991)

Table 9. Concentration of Closantel in Tissues of Cattle (n=4/group) Treated with a Single Oral Dose of 10 mg/kg (ppm)

Withdrawal Time (days)	Muscle	Liver	Kidney	Fat
14	0.41±0.10	0.68±0.52	2.14±1.00	0.65±0.20
28	0.19±0.05[1]	0.16±0.02[1]	0.83±0.31	0.18±0.03[2]
42	0.19±0.10[2]	0.49[3]	0.33±0.26	ND

1 - This mean does not include two values which are ≤ 0.10 ppm.
2 - This mean does not include one value which is ≤ 0.10 ppm.
3 - This mean does not include three values which are ≤ 0.10 ppm.
ND - All values are ≤ 0.10 ppm.

Two groups of six calves, mean body weight 118 ± 22 kg, were injected intramuscularly with closantel at 2.5 mg/kg. A group of three animals was sacrificed at 56 and 84 days after treatment. Samples of liver, kidney, muscle and fat were taken for analysis of closantel. Blood samples were collected from all animals every two weeks up to the time of sacrifice. Closantel was determined with an HPLC procedure having a 0.1 ppm detection limit.

The concentration of closantel in plasma averaged 10 ppm at 14 days. The $t_{1/2}$ for the elimination of closantel from plasma was ~12 days. By 70 days after treatment, closantel was mostly undetectable in plasma. Residues of closantel were not detected in any tissue at 56 days. (Michiels et al., 1980a)

Five groups of three steers, body weight ~200 kg, were treated subcutaneously with closantel according to the schedule below:

Treatment Day	Dose (mg/kg)	Sampling Day	Sample
0	15		
21	15	21	plasma
		35	plasma + tissue
50	10		
		65	plasma + tissue
80	10		
		95	tissue
120	10		
		135	plasma + tissue
		150	tissue

Blood samples were obtained on EDTA from the three animals of the last surviving group at the time of the second injection and further at 2 weeks after the second, third and fifth dose. Groups of three animals were sacrificed at 2 weeks after each injection beginning from the second dose and at four weeks after the last dose. Samples of edible tissues were collected for analysis of closantel with the HPLC method. The sampling scheme is summarized in the chart above.

Plasma concentrations of closantel ranged between 88 and 150 ppm for the period of drug administration. The results of the tissue residue analyses are summarized in Table 10. Highest levels of closantel were observed in the kidneys of treated steers. (Michiels et al., 1980b)

Table 10. Mean Tissue Concentrations of Closantel in Steers After Multiple Administration (ppm)

Tissue	Closantel Concentration on Day of Experiment 35	65	95	135	150
muscle-psoas	8.47	6.69	4.99	5.25	2.94
muscle-semitendinosus	4.36	4.15	3.84	2.79	2.82
liver	15.6	14.6	14.1	15.7	10.3
kidney	20.5	19.7	20.1	19.4	12.7
fat-subcutaneous	7.65	7.51	9.04	10.1	2.48
fat-perirenal	3.55	6.29	5.77	11.2	4.56

Four female and six male calves averaging 166 kg were injected intramuscularly with closantel at 2.5 mg/kg. Groups of three animals (1 F, 2 MA) were sacrificed at 14, 28 and 42 days of withdrawal. Samples of muscle, liver, kidney and perirenal fat were taken for analysis. A serum sample was taken from one animal of each group and from one surviving female at 56 days of withdrawal. Closantel was determined using an HPLC method having a detection limit of 0.1 ppm.

The results of this study are shown in Table 11. Highest concentrations of closantel were seen initially in kidney. Very little, if any, depletion of closantel occurred in the edible tissues of calves over the first 28 days of withdrawal. In fact, over the time period studied the concentration of closantel in fat seemed to increase slightly. (Michiels et al., 1979)

Table 11. Concentration of Closantel in Tissues of Calves Treated with a Single Intramuscular Dose of 2.5 mg/kg (ppm)

Withdrawal Time (days)	Muscle	Liver	Kidney	Fat	Serum
14	0.67	1.54	2.84	2.08	21
28	0.70	1.43	2.93	1.97	13
42	0.29	0.56	1.39	2.36	9
56	NA	NA	NA	NA	6.8

Five male and two female calves averaging 203 kg were injected intramuscularly with closantel at 5 mg/kg. A group of three animals (2 MA, 1 F) were sacrificed at 28 and 56 days of withdrawal. Samples of edible tissues were taken for analysis. A serum sample was taken from one female at 28 days and one male at 84 days of withdrawal. Analyses for closantel were done with an HPLC procedure (detection limit, 0.1 ppm).

The results of this experiment are presented in Table 12. The data for this study, in contrast those in Table 11, show depletion of closantel in fat. (Michiels et al., 1979)

Table 12. Concentration of Closantel in Tissues of Calves Treated with a Single Intramuscular Dose of 5 mg/kg (ppm)

Withdrawal Time (days)	Muscle	Liver	Kidney	Fat	Serum
28	0.94	1.71	4.95	6.03	20
56	0.39	0.58	1.58	1.31	NA
84	NA	NA	NA	NA	2.3

Three dairy cows, average weight 350 kg, were treated with a single intramuscular dose of closantel at 5 mg/kg. Milk and blood were taken at various times post dose. Samples were examined for closantel using HPLC with UV detection (limit of detection, ~0.5 ppm). Plasma concentrations of closantel were highest 1 to 5 days post dose, ranging ~44-45 ppm. After 5 days, closantel depleted from plasma with a $t_{1/2}$ of ~12 days. The depletion of closantel from milk is shown in Table 13. Mean concentrations of closantel in milk peaked at 4 to 7 days post dose. (Michiels et al., 1977b)

Table 13. Mean Concentrations of Closantel in Milk of Three Dairy Cows After a Single Intramuscular Dose at 5 mg/kg (ppm)

Time (days)	Concentration
1	0.47
2	0.80
3	0.66
4	1.01
5	0.88
6	0.92
7	1.07
14	0.48
21	0.52
28	0.08
35	0.22

METHODS OF ANALYSIS FOR RESIDUES IN TISSUES

Gas liquid chromatographic (GLC) and high pressure liquid chromatographic (HPLC) methods have been investigated for the determination of closantel in plasma and tissues of treated animals.

A GLC procedure for closantel in plasma and tissues of sheep has been developed. The method involves extraction of the sample, silylation of closantel and added internal standard, and analysis using electron capture detection. The limit of detection is 0.1 ppm. Continuous use of this method in analyzing tissue samples yielded a number of difficulties, including the appearance of interference peaks and a severe decrease in the sensitivity of the electron capture detector. (Woestenborghs et al., 1977; Woestenborghs et al., 1979)

The earliest investigations with HPLC for the determination of closantel led to a procedure for plasma of sheep. In this method, samples, to which an internal standard has been added, are extracted and then analyzed using HPLC with UV detection. The detection limit is ~0.5 ppm. (Hendrickx et al., 1976)

An HPLC procedure was developed for closantel in animal tissues as well as plasma using improved extraction techniques. In this method samples to which internal standard has been added are extracted with a SEP-PAK™ C18 cartridge. Following separation with HPLC, the samples are quantified using UV detection. The limit of detection is 0.1 ppm. (Woestenborghs et al., 1979)

The HPLC method above was modified to make the determination of closantel in plasma at levels exceeding 1 ppm more convenient. In the new procedure, sample containing internal standard is deproteinated and then analyzed using HPLC with UV detection. No separate purification step is necessary. (Woestenborghs et al., 1985)

APPRAISAL

The depletion of residues of closantel from the edible tissues of sheep and cattle has been studied using radiolabelled and unlabeled drug.

The characteristics of residue depletion in the edible tissues of cattle and sheep that have been treated with closantel are similar. In particular, residues of the parent drug are highest in kidney over the entire range of the withdrawal periods studied (usually to 56 days); the residues deplete from tissues with a $t_{1/2}$ normally in the 2-3 week range; in sheep, the parenteral and the oral routes of administration yield comparable residue concentrations when the oral dose is twice the parenteral dose (an oral dose is roughly 50% as bioavailable as the parenteral dose).

From the studies in which sheep were treated either orally or parenterally with radiolabelled closantel, it was found that parent closantel accounted for nearly all the total radioactivity in muscle, fat and kidney; i.e., virtually no metabolism occurs in those tissues. In sheep liver, approximately 60-70% of the radioactivity was parent closantel, with the remaining residue being comprised of 3- and 5-monoiodoclosantel. No evidence for alternate metabolic pathways (e.g., amide hydrolysis or complete deiodination) was reported. In cattle treated orally, parent closantel accounts for approximately 100, 80 and 70 % of the total residues in muscle, kidney and fat, respectively. However, in cattle liver approximately 10% of the radioactivity was parent closantel, and 40-77% of the radioactivity was accounted for by 3-monoiodoclosantel. In addition, a metabolite accounting for 6% of the radioactivity was identified as a sulfate conjugate of a closantel-derivative. No radiolabelled studies have been conducted with closantel administered parenterally in cattle.

The metabolism work in rats demonstrates a similarity with that in sheep and cattle. It appears that metabolites present in the edible tissues of sheep and cattle are produced as well in rats. The only exception is the small amount of the sulfate conjugate metabolite in cattle. In addition, the presence of deiodinated closantel and monoiodosalicylic acid is reported in rats.

Of particular interest from the standpoint of residue monitoring, the depletion of residues of closantel from plasma parallels that from the edible tissues. That is, there is a fairly constant tissue:plasma ratio within species which is independent of time (see Tables 3 and 5). The extrapolation of concentrations of closantel residues from plasma to edible tissues therefore seems feasible. By extension, the monitoring of plasma may then be of potential use in determining when treated animals may be marketed.

JECFA used the residue chemistry data in the monograph developed for the 36th Session of JECFA to recommend MRLs in sheep. However, since the last meeting it has been recognized that the MRL calculation of 1.5 ppm for kidney at 28 days may be exceeded at that time due to the concentrations of parent closantel in the oral radiolabelled study in sheep at 35 and 42 days (Meuldermans et al., 1982). Therefore, the MRL has been reevaluated and determined that an increase to 5 ppm in kidney will not impact the drug's human food safety. This change has been incorporated in Table 14.

Sheep - Based on the ADI of 0-0.03 mg/kg established by the 36th Meeting of JECFA, the permitted daily intake of closantel would be 1.8 mg of total drug-related residue contributed by 500 g of food animal meat in the diet of a 60-kg person. For all dose levels studied in sheep, the ADI is not exceeded at 14 days. The doses studied were 10 mg/kg orally or 5 mg/kg intramuscularly. At 28 days of withdrawal, the intake of residues of closantel is well below the ADI. Based on the data from the studies using closantel at 10 mg/kg orally and 5 mg/kg intramuscularly, JECFA recommended an MRL of 5000 μg/kg for parent closantel in kidney and 1500 μg/kg in muscle and liver and 2000 μg/kg in fat of sheep. See Table 14.

Table 14. Recommended MRLs μg/kg for Closantel in Sheep

	Observed Concentration at Day 28 Withdrawal, mg/kg		mg Closantel Consumed			
Tissue	10 mg/kg Oral	5 mg/kg IM	Oral	IM	Rec. MRL (parent)	mg(a) Consumed (Theory)
Muscle	<0.4	1.1	0.12	0.33	1500	0.45
Liver	0.8(1.14)b	0.7(1.17)c	0.11	0.12	1500 (2500)c	0.25
Kidney	0.7	1.2	0.04	0.06	5000	0.25
Fat	0.7	0.4	0.04	0.02	2000	0.10
Total			0.31	0.53		1.05

a) Based on a daily intake of 0.3 kg muscle, 0.1 kg liver, 0.05 kg kidney and fat.
b) Adjusted observed value by 70% to estimate total residues.
c) Adjusted observed value by 60% to estimate total residues.

Cattle - Temporary MRLs in cattle were proposed at the 36th Session of JECFA, but based on the development of a more complete residue package for cattle having been submitted, the Committee recommends the new MRLs. At 42 days of withdrawal, the intake of residues of closantel is below the ADI of 1.8 mg. Based on the data from the studies using closantel at 10 mg/kg orally and 2.5 mg/kg intramuscularly, JECFA recommended an MRL of 1000 μg/kg for parent closantel in muscle and liver, and 3000 μg/kg in kidney and fat (see Table 15).

Table 15. Recommended MRLs μg/kg for Closantel in Cattle

Tissue	Observed Concentration at Day 28* or 42* Withdrawal, mg/kg		mg Closantel Consumed			
	10 mg/kg Oral	2.5 mg/kg IM	Oral	IM	Rec. MRL (parent)	mg(a) Consumed (Theory)
Muscle	0.19	0.29	0.06	0.09	1000	0.30
Liver	0.16(1.6)b	0.56(5.6)b	0.16	0.56	1000(10000)b	1.00
Kidney	0.83(1.0)c	1.39(1.7)c	0.05	0.09	3000(3750)c	0.19
Fat	0.7(1.0)d	2.36(3.4)d	0.05	0.17	3000(4290)d	0.21
Total			0.32	0.91		1.70

* - The oral data is summarized from Day 28 withdrawal and the parenteral data is summarized from Day 42 withdrawal.

a) Based on a daily intake of 0.3 kg muscle, 0.1 kg liver, 0.05 kg kidney and fat.

b) Adjusted observed value by 10% to estimate total residues.

c) Adjusted observed value by 80% to estimate total residues.

d) Adjusted observed value by 70% to estimate total residues.

REFERENCES

Hendrickx, J., Wynants, J. and Heykants, J. 1976. A "HPLC" assay method for closantel (R 31520) in sheep plasma. Unpublished report V 2710. Submitted to FAO by Janssen Pharmaceutica, B-2340 Beerse, Belgium.

Mannens, G., Mostmans, E., Verboven, P., Hendrickx, J., Hurkmans, R., Van Leemput, L., Meuldermans, W. and Heykants, J. 1989. The excretion and metabolism of ^{14}C-closantel in male Wistar rats after a single oral dose of 10 mg/kg. Unpublished report V 7201. Submitted to FAO by Janssen Pharmaceutica, B-2340 Beerse, Belgium.

Meuldermans, W., Michiels, M., Woestenborghs, R., Van Houdt, J., Lorreyne, W., Hendrickx, J., Heykants, J. and Desplenter, L. 1982. Absorption, tissue distribution, excretion and metabolism of closantel-^{14}C after intramuscular and oral administration in sheep. Unpublished report V 4523. Submitted to FAO by Janssen Pharmaceutica, B-2340 Beerse, Belgium.

Michiels, M., Woestenborghs, R., Heykants, J. and Marsboom, R. 1977a. On the absorption and distribution of closantel (R 31520) in sheep after oral and intramuscular administration. Unpublished report V 2709. Submitted to FAO by Janssen Pharmaceutica, B-2340 Beerse, Belgium.

Michiels, M., Hendrickx, J., Heykants, J. and Marsboom, R. 1977b. Plasma and milk concentrations of closantel in cattle after a single intramuscular administration. Unpublished report V 2706. Submitted to FAO by Janssen Pharmaceutica, B-2340 Beerse, Belgium.

Michiels, M., Woestenborghs, R., Michielsen, L., Hendrickx, J., Heykants, J. and Marsboom, R. 1979. Residual plasma and tissue concentrations of closantel (R 31520) in cattle and sheep. Unpublished report V 3173. Submitted to FAO by Janssen Pharmaceutica, B-2340 Beerse, Belgium.

Michiels, M., Woestenborghs, R., Embrechts, L., Heykants, J. and Marsboom, R. 1980a. Plasma levels and residual tissue concentrations of closantel (R 31520) in sheep and cattle. Unpublished report V 3413. Submitted to FAO by Janssen Pharmaceutica, B-2340 Beerse, Belgium.

Michiels, M., Woestenborghs, R., Embrechts, L., Heykants, J. and Marsboom, R. 1980b. Residual plasma and tissue concentrations of closantel (R 31520) in cattle. Unpublished report V 3716. Submitted to FAO by Janssen Pharmaceutica, B-2340 Beerse, Belgium.

Michiels, M., Meuldermans, W. and Heykants, J. 1987. The metabolism and fate of closantel (Flukiver) in sheep and cattle. Drug Metab. Rev., **18**, 235-251.

Van Beijsterveldt, L., Van Leemput, L. and Heykants, J. 1991. Closantel: tissue residues in cattle after single oral treatment at 10 mg/kg with a 5 % suspension formulation. Unpublished report V 7865. Submitted to FAO by Janssen Pharmaceutica, B-2340 Beerse, Belgium.

Van Beijsterveldt, L., Van Leemput, L., Woestenborghs, R., Meuldermans, W. and Heykants, J. 1989. Serum levels of closantel in the male Wistar rat after single oral administration at 20 mg/kg. Unpublished report V 7202. Submitted to FAO by Janssen Pharmaceutica, B-2340 Beerse, Belgium.

Van Leemput, L. and Heykants, J. 1991. Absorption, tissue distribution, excretion and metabolism of ^{14}C-closantel in cattle after a single oral dose of 10 mg/kg. Unpublished report V 7864. Submitted to FAO by Janssen Pharmaceutica, B-2340 Beerse, Belgium.

Woestenborghs, R., Hendrickx, J., Michiels, M., Michielsen, L. and Heykants, J. 1979. A new HPLC-method for the determination of closantel (R 31520) in plasma and animal tissues. Unpublished report V 3190. Submitted to FAO by Janssen Pharmaceutica, B-2340 Beerse, Belgium.

Woestenborghs, R., Hendrickx, J., Michiels, M., Michielsen, L. and Heykants, J. 1985. A modified HPLC-method for the rapid determination of closantel in animal plasma. Unpublished report V 5907. Submitted to FAO by Janssen Pharmaceutica, B-2340 Beerse, Belgium.

Woestenborghs, R., Michiels, M. and Heykants, J. 1977. Electron capture GLC determination of closantel (R 31520) in plasma and animal tissues. Unpublished report V 2708. Submitted to FAO by Janssen Pharmaceutica, B-2340 Beerse, Belgium.

FLUBENDAZOLE

IDENTITY

Chemical name: Flubendazole

CAS Number: 31430-15-6

CAS Nomenclature: [5-(4-Fluorobenzoyl)-1H-benzimidazol-2-yl]carbamic acid methyl ester

Synonyms: Fluvermal, Flubenol, Flumoxal, Flumoxane

Structural formula:

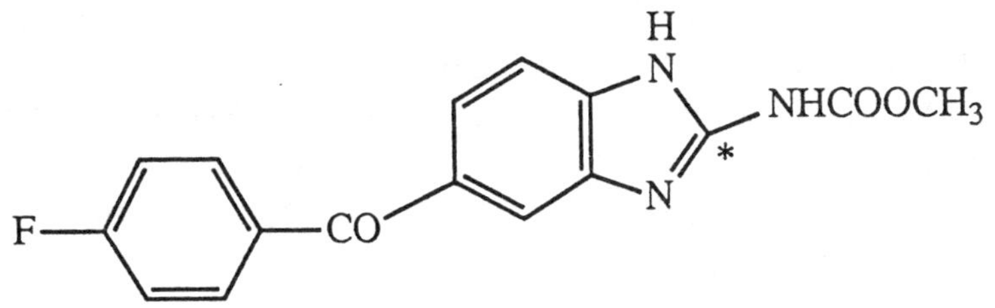

(* shows position of ^{14}C label for metabolism studies)

Molecular formula: $C_{16}H_{12}FN_3O_3$

Molecular weight: 313.30

OTHER INFORMATION ON IDENTITY AND PROPERTIES

Pure active ingredient: Flubendazole active ingredient contains not less than 95.0% of $C_{16}H_{12}FN_3O_3$, calculated on a dry basis.

Appearance: Grey-white to yellowish powder.

Melting point: 260°C

Solubility: Flubendazole is almost insoluble in water and most common organic solvents [diluted mineral acids, ethanol, ether, chloroform (0.014 g/100 ml)]. It is fairly soluble in formic acid (34.05 g/100 ml).

RESIDUES IN FOOD AND THEIR EVALUATION

CONDITIONS OF USE

General

Flubendazole is a member of a widely used chemical class of compounds known as the benzimidazoles. Its chemical structure and pharmacological properties are similar to other benzimidazoles such as thiabendazole, fenbendazole, oxibendazole, mebendazole, oxfendazole and triclabendazole.

Flubendazole is a broad-spectrum anthelmintic used for deworming dogs, cats, swine, and poultry. It is active against gastrointestinal nematodes and lungworms in swine and against gastrointestinal nematodes in poultry. For therapeutic treatment, pigs are given feed containing 30 g flubendazole per ton (30 ppm) of feed for 10 consecutive days. For poultry, the following treatments are recommended for 7 consecutive days: 20 g per ton (20 ppm) of feed for turkeys, 30 or 60 g per ton (30 or 60 ppm) for chickens and geese; and 60 g per ton (60 ppm) for pheasants and partridges. For disease prevention, chickens may be treated continuously with feed containing 4 g per ton (4 ppm) flubendazole.

Dosages

Flubendazole is administered as a feed additive to swine and poultry, or orally as a paste (44 mg/ml) to dogs and cats. Because of poor solubility in aqueous systems, the drug is suitable for oral administration and generally is not available for parenteral treatment.

METABOLISM

General

The absorption, distribution, metabolism, excretion and tissue residues of flubendazole have been studied using ^{14}C-labeled drug in rats, dogs, swine, and poultry. In all studies where the radioactive label site was identified, the molecule was labeled in the 2-position of the benzimidazole ring, as shown in the chemical structure above. Flubendazole is poorly absorbed and the metabolism is qualitatively similar in all species studied. Efficacy against gastrointestinal parasites has been attributed to the poor bioavailability of flubendazole, causing most of the drug to be eliminated in the feces as unchanged flubendazole. The portion of drug that becomes absorbed is rapidly metabolized, resulting in extremely low levels of parent drug in blood or urine. The major metabolites in urine of all species result from carbamate hydrolysis or ketone reduction. Metabolites were present in urine mainly as glucuronide or sulphate conjugates.

When swine or poultry are treated with flubendazole, the tissue with the highest residue concentration and slowest depletion rate is the liver. The major metabolite in swine liver is (2-amino-1H-benzimidazol-5-yl) 4-fluorophenyl-methanone. This compound is found at a much higher concentration than parent flubendazole and could serve as a marker residue. Residues were higher and more persistent in egg yolk than egg white.

The rat and dog are exposed to nearly the same metabolites that are present in the edible tissues of swine. One minor metabolite found in the dog was not reported in swine or rats. This compound, 2-amino-α-(4-fluorophenyl)-1-methyl-1H-benzimidazole-5-methanol (Compound (5) in Figure 1), resulted from N-methylation. Metabolism information was not available for poultry. However, a radiolabeled residue depletion study included information on excretion. Rate of excretion in poultry was similar to that of rats and dogs. Of the total radioactive dose, 86 to 87% was excreted as unchanged drug within 24 hours of the last treatment. Absorption of flubendazole may be greater in swine than in rats and dogs. In swine, only 79% of the total radioactive dose had been excreted by the end of the 30 day withdrawal period. Within 4 days post-dosing, 96% and 88% of the total radioactive dose had been excreted by rats and dogs, respectively.

Rat

Twenty-four male Wistar rats (250 ± 10 g) were treated orally with a microcrystalline suspension of ^{14}C-flubendazole. The rats received a 10 mg/kg dose with specific activity of 2.03 μCi/mg (radiochemical purity and label position not-specified). Plasma levels of unchanged flubendazole reached 0.130 μg/ml one-half hour after treatment. In plasma, total drug related residue peaked at 0.504 μg/ml eight hours after treatment. The elimination half life was approximately 6 hours for unchanged drug, measured by HPLC with UV detection at 313 nm. Plasma clearance of labeled metabolites was much slower. At 24 hours post-treatment, approximately 50% of the total radioactive dose had been eliminated in the feces, primarily as unchanged flubendazole. Only about 4% of the total radioactive dose was excreted in the urine by 24 hours, all as metabolites. (Michiels et al., 1977a)

In a study comparing the excretion and metabolism of flubendazole and mebendazole, flubendazole was given to five male Wistar rats (275 to 285 g) at 10 mg/kg. Dosing was by oral injection with a microcrystalline suspension of ^{14}C-flubendazole labeled in the 2-position. The drug was radiochemically pure (exact purity not-stated) when tested by TLC, and had a specific activity of 6.7 μCi/mg. A high percentage of the total radioactive dose was recovered in the excreta within four days (89% feces, 7% urine) after treatment. Unchanged drug was measured using HPLC with detection at 254 nm. Metabolites were identified by TLC, comparing purified urine and fecal extracts with reference compounds. Radioactivity in the feces was almost entirely from unchanged drug, but urinary ^{14}C was primarily from metabolites. The main metabolite in feces and urine resulted from carbamate hydrolysis. In addition, another metabolic pathway was reduction of the ketone, resulting in additional metabolites in urine (Figure 1). The major metabolites in urine were unchanged flubendazole (9.8% of 0 to 48 h radioactivity in urine), methyl-[5-(α-hydroxy-α-(4-fluorophenyl) methyl)-1H-benzimidazol-2-yl] carbamate (19.0%), and (2-amino-1H-benzimidazol-5-yl) 4-fluorophenyl-methanone (15.8%). Another peak amounting to 15.8% of total radioactivity could not be identified. In feces, 87.3% of the 0 to 24 hour radioactivity was from unchanged drug and 2.5% from (2-amino-1H-benzimidazol-5-yl) 4-fluorophenyl-methanone. (Meuldermans et al., 1977)

A study was conducted to compare the absorption of flubendazole in Wistar and multimammate rats. Rats received an oral dose of 40 mg/kg ^{14}C-flubendazole. Treatment groups included 18 Wistar or 12 multimammate rats. Plasma levels of flubendazole measured by radioimmunoassay, reached 81 ng/ml by 4 hours after oral administration to Wistar rats. In the multimammate rats, plasma concentrations were approximately 4 times lower than in Wistar rats. Substantial differences in drug absorption were observed in these two rat strains. (Michiels et al., 1980)

Dog

A 10 mg/kg oral dose of ^{14}C-flubendazole (labeled in 2-position) was given to three female Beagle dogs (weight 12.0, 13.2, and 14.2 kg). The ^{14}C-flubendazole (specific activity of 0.76 μCi/mg) was radiochemically pure when tested by TLC and inverse isotope dilution techniques. Plasma levels of total radioactivity reached a maximum of 0.23 μg/ml flubendazole equivalents at 24 hours post-dosing. Unchanged drug in plasma, measured by HPLC with detection at 313 nm, was below the detection limit of 0.01 μg/ml throughout the 96 hour post-treatment sampling period. About 88% of the total radioactive dose was excreted within four days, 81.5% with the feces and 6.3% in the urine. More than 90% of the radioactivity in the feces was from parent drug. Radioactivity in the urine was almost entirely from metabolites. Metabolites were characterized by HPLC with UV detection at 247 nm, MS, and NMR. The main metabolic pathways were the same for the dog as for the rat. These were reduction of the ketone and hydrolysis of the carbamate. The resulting basic metabolites were mainly present in urine as glucuronide or sulphate conjugates. In the dog, a novel (although minor) metabolite was detected, identified tentatively as 2-amino-α-(4-fluorophenyl)-1-methyl-1H-benzimidazole-5-methanol (compound (5) in Figure 1). (Meuldermans et al., 1978)

Swine

Metabolism in swine was studied using eighteen feeder pigs (weight 16.7 to 24.5 kg) treated orally with ^{14}C-flubendazole at 1.5 mg/kg daily for five consecutive days (total dose 7.5 mg/kg). This dose level was given to simulate treatment with 30 ppm flubendazole in the feed. The test substance, labeled in the 2-position of the benzimidazole ring, had a specific activity of 9.25 μCi/mg. The radio and chemical purity of the test compound was not-specified. Thirty days after the end of the medication period, 79% of the administered dose had been excreted, 23% with the urine and 56% with the feces. Metabolite analysis required first extracting tissue samples with methanol and water. Samples were cleaned up using Sep-Pak C_{18} cartridges and then analyzed by reverse phase HPLC with a radioactivity detector. The major metabolites in swine feces and urine were the same as for rats and dogs. The main urinary metabolite resulted from both carbamate hydrolysis and ketone reduction (compound (4) in Figure 1). In feces, the main metabolite was from carbamate hydrolysis (compound (3) in Figure 1). In tissues, the major metabolites were the same as those found in urine and feces. The major metabolite in swine liver was (2-amino-1H-benzimidazol-5-yl) 4-fluorophenyl-methanone (compound (3) in Figure 1). This metabolite might be suitable for regulatory monitoring. Actual numerical values for metabolite concentrations were not included in this report. When extrapolated from a graph at zero withdrawal, approximately 1.5 ppm or one-third of total residue in liver was the metabolite (3) in Figure 1. Unchanged flubendazole levels were approximately 0.06 ppm or less than 2% of total residue. In kidney, similar ratios were found between total residue, parent flubendazole, and this metabolite (3). (Meuldermans et al., 1982)

TISSUE RESIDUE DEPLETION STUDIES

Radiolabeled Residue Depletion Studies

Rat

The following residue data were from one of the metabolism studies discussed above. Three rats were slaughtered at each time listed in Table 1, which includes a summary of total residues (TR) and unchanged flubendazole (UD) in plasma and tissues. Total residues were highest in liver and kidney during the 24 hour testing period. Unchanged drug is a minor proportion of total residue in all tissues except fat. In fat, UD represented 6% of TR at 1 hour and more than 100% at 6 hours withdrawal. (Michiels et al., 1977a)

Table 1. Total residue (TR) and Unchanged Flubendazole (UD) in Wistar rats after oral dosing at 10 mg/kg.

Time	Plasma		Liver		Kidney		Muscle		Fat	
(h)	(μg/ml)				(μg/g)					
	TR	UD	TR	UD	TR	UD	TR	UD	TR	UD
0.5	0.309	0.130	1.61	0.016	1.38	0.039	0.197	NG*	0.239	NG
1	0.304	0.110	1.90	0.015	1.65	0.028	0.253	0.080	0.793	0.049
2	0.223	0.076	1.67	0.034	1.75	0.05	0.202	0.066	0.465	0.283
4	0.363	0.085	1.78	0.018	1.77	0.062	0.198	0.048	0.277	0.186
6	0.449	0.083	2.68	0.014	2.99	0.032	0.312	0.050	0.227	0.250
8	0.504	0.071	2.84	≤0.01	3.09	0.041	0.296	0.034	0.223	0.120
16	0.278	0.011	1.68	<0.01	0.881	<0.01	0.129	NG	0.164	0.068
24	0.296	≤0.01	1.29	<0.01	1.29	0.022	0.111	NG	0.140	0.039

*NG = No value given.

Swine

A radiolabeled residue depletion study was conducted using the same eighteen pigs used for the metabolism study described above. Dosing information is included in the section above on metabolism. Data for the total residue portion of the metabolism study in swine tissue (see above) are summarized in Table 2. At each withdrawal time, values are means from three pigs. Total residues were highest in liver throughout the 30 day withdrawal period. (Meuldermans et al., 1982); (Lee, 1981)

Table 2. Total Residues of ^{14}C-Flubendazole in Swine Tissue (ppb ± SD).

Withdrawal Time	Liver	Kidney	Muscle	Fat
6 hours	3865 ± 1046	2678 ± 488	262 ± 69	212 ± 94
5 days	1863 ± 1453	435 ± 448	35.5 ± 34.9	50.1 ± 52.3
10 days	529 ± 212	78.2 ± 23.0	10.5 ± 4.8	16.3 ± 9.0
16 days	433 ± 66	76.6 ± 44.3	8.66 ± 4.29	15.6 ± 10.0
23 days	194 ± 85	49.9 ± 23.8	8.67 ± 2.74	13.5 ± 7.2
30 days	106 ± 44	22.5 ± 6.2	2.51 ± 0.32	3.38 ± 0.92

Poultry

Twenty-eight laying hens (average weight 3.6 kg, 34 weeks old) received gelatin capsules containing ^{14}C-flubendazole at a dose equivalent to 30 ppm in the food for seven consecutive days. Flubendazole was labeled in the 2-position of the benzimidazole ring. Drug with a radiochemical purity of 98.5% was mixed with unlabeled flubendazole to give a final specific activity of about 8 μCi/mg. At all withdrawal times tested from 1 to 14 days post-treatment, radioactive equivalents of flubendazole in blood and plasma were less than 0.01 μg/ml, suggesting that absorption was poor. Within 24 hours of the final dose, 86 to 87% of the administered radioactivity had been excreted, primarily as unchanged flubendazole. After total radioactivity levels reached steady state in 5 to 6 days, eggs contained an average of 0.11 to 0.12 μg equivalents flubendazole/g. Radioactivity in the yolks was much higher than in the egg white. The highest observed levels of radioactivity in tissue were 0.21 μg equivalents/g in liver and 0.08 μg/g in kidney at 24 hours past the last dose. Table 3 includes a summary of total radioactive residues of flubendazole in eggs and Table 4 summarizes residues in plasma and tissue. Days 0 through 6 are on treatment and 7 through twenty represent the withdrawal period. (Michiels et al., 1983)

Table 3. Total Residue of Flubendazole μg/g (SD) in Eggs.

Time (days)	Egg White	Egg Yolk	Total Egg
0	≤0.001	≤0.001	≤0.001
1	0.016 (0.009)	0.030 (0.012)	0.020 (0.009)
2	0.014 (0.008)	0.048 (0.033)	0.026 (0.016)
3	0.017 (0.009)	0.098 (0.058)	0.045 (0.024)
4	0.017 (0.006)	0.184 (0.062)	0.073 (0.024)
5	0.020 (0.008)	0.279 (0.082)	0.109 (0.033)
6	0.018 (0.010)	0.294 (0.120)	0.116 (0.048)
7	0.015 (0.006)	0.306 (0.078)	0.117 (0.031)
8	0.009 (0.008)	0.309 (0.103)	0.115 (0.043)
9	0.004 (0.003)	0.339 (0.098)	0.121 (0.038)
10	0.002 (0.001)	0.268 (0.088)	0.095 (0.032)
11	≤0.001	0.220 (0.091)	0.077 (0.036)
12	≤0.001	0.161 (0.076)	0.059 (0.034)
13	≤0.001	0.117 (0.053)	0.041 (0.020)
14	≤0.001	0.074 (0.050)	0.031 (0.018)
15	≤0.001	0.026 (0.026)	0.010 (0.009)
16	≤0.001	0.010 (0.010)	0.003 (0.004)
17	≤0.001	0.004 (0.004)	≤0.001
18	≤0.001	≤0.001	≤0.001
19	≤0.001	≤0.001	≤0.001
20	≤0.001	≤0.001	≤0.001

Table 4. Total Residues of Flubendazole μg/ml or g (SD) in Tissues and Plasma of Laying Hens.

Study day (withdrawal day)	Plasma	Liver	Kidney	Muscle	Fat
7 (1)	0.007 (0.002)	0.210 (0.047)	0.080 (0.044)	≤0.01	≤0.01
8 (2)	0.005 (0.003)	0.146 (0.032)	0.054 (0.028)	≤0.01	≤0.01
10 (4)	0.002 (0.001)	0.069 (0.026)	0.010 (0.001)	≤0.01	≤0.01
13 (7)	0.001 (0.000)	0.073 (0.033)	≤0.01	≤0.01	≤0.01
17 (11)	≤0.001	0.030 (0.013)	≤0.01	≤0.01	≤0.01
20 (14)	≤0.001	0.016 (0.013)	≤0.01	≤0.01	≤0.01

OTHER RESIDUE DEPLETION STUDIES

Residue Depletion Studies with Unlabeled Drug

Swine

Three male pigs (20 to 25 kg) received flubendazole at 30 ppm in the feed for five consecutive days. Flubendazole levels measured by HPLC (UV detection at 254 nm) were less than 0.01 µg/g (method sensitivity) in plasma, liver, kidney, muscle, and fat at all slaughter times of 16, 30, and 54 hours withdrawal. In an additional study, seven sows (weight 121 to 163 kg) were treated with feed containing 30 ppm flubendazole for ten consecutive days. At 30 ppm in feed, the sows received about 0.5 mg/kg body weight per day. The sows were slaughtered at seven days after the last treatment with flubendazole. Mean levels of flubendazole were 0.059, 0.067, 0.013, and 0.033 µg/g for liver, kidney, muscle, and fat, respectively. (Michiels et al., 1976)

When a single dose of 5 mg flubendazole (by capsule) per kg was given to three male pigs (20 to 25 kg), measurable residues were detected in fat. Analysis by HPLC with UV detection at 313 nm showed 0.06, 0.06, and 0.07 µg/g flubendazole in fat at 24, 48, and 72 hours withdrawal, respectively. Residues in muscle and liver were 0.01 µg/g (method sensitivity) or less at all slaughter times. In kidney, 0.02 µg/g flubendazole was determined at 48 and 72 hours withdrawal. These data are summarized in Table 5 below (one animal per slaughter time). (Michiels et al., 1977b)

Table 5. Flubendazole µg/ml or g (SD not given) in Swine Tissue after a Single Oral Dose

Withdrawal Time (h)	Plasma	Liver	Kidney	Muscle	Fat
24	0.02	<0.01	<0.01	<0.01	0.06
48	0.03	0.01	0.02	<0.01	0.06
72	<0.01	0.01	0.02	0.01	0.07

Another residue study was conducted using single 5 mg/kg dosing in three groups of five male pigs (weight 20 to 25 kg). Tissues and plasma were analyzed using a radioimmunoassay (RIA) with quantitation limits of 1 ppb in plasma and 5 ppb in tissue. Animals were slaughtered in groups of five at 24, 72, and 168 hours after dosing. Slightly higher levels of flubendazole in tissue were found in this study with a single 5 mg/kg dose than when pigs received 30 ppm in the feed for 5 days. The difference in results could be attributed to either the dosing method or differences in the analytical method (RIA vs HPLC). Results are summarized in Table 6. (Michiels et al., 1979)

Table 6. Flubendazole μg/ml or g (SD) in Swine Tissue after a Single Oral Dose

Withdrawal Time (h)	Plasma	Liver	Kidney	Muscle	Fat
24	<0.001	0.12 (0.16)	0.12 (0.16)	0.07 (0.05)	0.10 (0.08)
72	<0.001	0.03 (0.01)	0.02 (0.01)	0.02 (0.01)	0.07 (0.03)
168	<0.001	≤0.005	≤0.005	0.01 (0.0)	0.02 (0.01)

Poultry

When chickens (number not stated) were treated with 60 ppm flubendazole for 7 days, residues were detectable in egg yolk for 11 days after treatment ended. Residues were higher in yolk than white. Eggs and tissues were analyzed using an HPLC method (detection method not-specified) that was sensitive to 0.010 μg/g. Of the tissues, liver had the greatest amount of residue at zero withdrawal, although flubendazole could not be detected in any tissue by 6 (n=1) and 7 (n=6) days withdrawal. Residue data are summarized in Table 7. (Tornoe and Christensen, undated)

Table 7. Residue μg/g (SD) in Chicken Tissue and Eggs after Treatment with feed containing 60 ppm flubendazole

Withdrawal Time, days	Egg Yolk	Egg White	Muscle	Kidney	Liver
0 (n=6)	0.592 (0.148)	0.036 (0.008)	0.079 (0.031)	0.173 (0.079)	0.198 (0.082)
4 (n=1)	NA	NA	0.071	0.236	0.200
6 (n=1)	NA	NA	ND	ND	ND
7 (n=6)	0.318 (0.128)	ND	ND	ND	ND
11 (n=6)	0.019 (0.010)	ND	NA	NA	NA
28 (n=6)	NA	NA	ND	ND	ND

Pheasants (20 males and 20 females) were treated with feed containing 60 ppm flubendazole for 7 consecutive days. Tissues and plasma were analyzed for flubendazole by HPLC with UV detection at 312 nm. Only skin with adhering fat contained measurable residues by 1 day of withdrawal. Results are summarized in Table 8. (Van Leemput and Heykants, 1991)

Table 8. Residues of Flubendazole in Pheasants. Values (ng/g) are Median of Ten Birds per Slaughter Time.

Withdrawal Time	Plasma	Liver	Kidney	Muscle	Skin/Fat
6 hours	16.5	35	57.5	18.5	76
1 day	≤10	≤10	≤10	≤10	29.5
4 days	≤10	≤10	≤10	≤10	22.5
7 days	≤10	≤10	≤10	≤10	12

METHODS OF ANALYSIS FOR RESIDUES IN TISSUES

Plasma and tissue levels of flubendazole in swine were measured using an HPLC method with UV detection at 313 nm. An internal standard, nocodazole, was added to plasma or tissue, followed by extracting twice with chloroform. The combined organic layers were dried, re-extracted several more times with organic solvents, and several pH adjustments were made. The final extracts were measured by HPLC. This method is sensitive to 0.01 ppm. (Michiels et al., 1977a)

A similar HPLC procedure with UV detection at 312 nm was used to measure flubendazole in plasma and tissue of pheasants. This procedure requires adding ammonium acetate and ammonia to samples, followed by extracting with a mixture of 95% heptane and 5% isoamyl alcohol. Extracts are dried and re-solubilized before analysis. The claimed detection limit is 0.01 μg/g. (Van Leemput and Heykants, 1991)

Another HPLC method was developed for flubendazole using UV detection at 254 nm. This procedure shows excellent separation between flubendazole and the major metabolite resulting from carbamate hydrolysis ((3) in Figure 1). The procedure was described for analysis of pure substances and did not include extraction procedures for tissues. (Fujisawa, 1981)

An HPLC method that has detection limits of 20 to 50 ppb has been developed for simultaneously determining eight benzimidazoles in meat. This method might be suitable for measuring flubendazole and the major metabolite found in swine tissue, (2-amino-1H-benzimidazol-5-yl) 4-fluorophenyl-methanone. Samples of ground tissue are homogenized with acetonitrile and then centrifuged. The supernatant was subjected to a series of organic extractions, followed by clean-up with Sep-Pak C_{18} and fluorosil cartridges. Solutions containing purified benzimidazoles were dried, re-dissolved, and assayed by HPLC using a reverse phase C_{18} column and UV detection at 298 nm. Individual benzimidazoles were confirmed using GC/MS. Before GC analysis, purified samples prepared for HPLC were used to form methyl and pentafluorobenzyl derivatives. Using spiked samples (0.1 μg/g), typical recoveries were above 70% for flubendazole in liver, kidney, or muscle. (Marti et al., 1990)

A radioimmunoassay (RIA), which was originally developed to measure mebendazole, was used to determine flubendazole in plasma and tissues. Mebendazole differs from flubendazole only by a fluorine substitution in the benzoyl portion of the molecule. Tissues were homogenized in a solution containing 10% formic acid in methanol. After centrifuging, a portion of the supernatant was added to control plasma, the antiserum, and ^{3}H-mebendazole. Following a 2 hour incubation at room temperature, a dextran-charcoal suspension was added to separate the bound and free drug. Samples were centrifuged again and radioactivity in the supernatant was determined by liquid scintillation counting. Radioactivity in the supernatant is from antibody-bound ^{3}H-mebendazole. Tissue concentrations were calculated using a standard curve prepared by adding flubendazole to control liver tissue. (Michiels et al., 1979)

The mebendazole antibodies used in the RIA procedure show a high degree of cross-reactivity with flubendazole, making it a suitable method for both drugs. Metabolites (2), (3), and (4) of Figure 1 did not bind well with the mebendazole antibodies. Thus the RIA assay would be reasonably specific for parent drug, but unlikely to measure other flubendazole related metabolites. (Michiels et al., 1978).

APPRAISAL

The following information was utilized in setting the MRLs for flubendazole:

An ADI of 0-12 μg/kg of body weight was established. This would result in a maximum ADI of 720 μg for a 60 kg human.

Assuming a total daily food intake from zero-withdrawal swine tissue (Table 2) and eggs (based on 30 mg/kg body weight study, Table 3), the daily intake of flubendazole-related residues would be 620 μg:

> {(3865 μg/kg x 0.1 kg of liver) + (2678 μg/kg x 0.05 kg of kidney) + (262 μg/kg x 0.3 kg of muscle) + (212 μg/kg x 0.05 kg of fat) + (120 μg/kg x 0.1 kg of egg)} = 620 μg

Eggs

The daily intake of flubendazole-related residues would likely remain below the ADI even when considering the large increase in residues in eggs resulting from the use of flubendazole at 60 mg/kg body weight. However, the argument that increased doses of flubendazole would not increase residue levels because of the low systemic availability appears not to be true for eggs. The levels of parent flubendazole in egg yolk from the 60 mg/kg body weight study are double the residue levels of all flubendazole-related residues from the 30 mg/kg body weight study.

A MRL for the whole egg of 400 μg/kg flubendazole is recommended.

Poultry

As no withdrawal period is required for poultry, parent flubendazole is an adequate marker residue.

MRLs of 500 and 200 µg/kg are recommended for poultry liver and muscle, respectively.

Swine

Although edible tissues from swine require no withdrawal period from a human food safety perspective, a withdrawal period will be used for swine based on good animal husbandry practices.

Parent flubendazole is a marginal marker residue for swine liver. However, methods are available for flubendazole and the residue data indicate that misuse will be detected by monitoring for parent flubendazole in swine tissue.

A MRL of 10 µg/kg is recommended for swine liver and muscle.

FIGURE 1
METABOLITES OF FLUBENDAZOLE

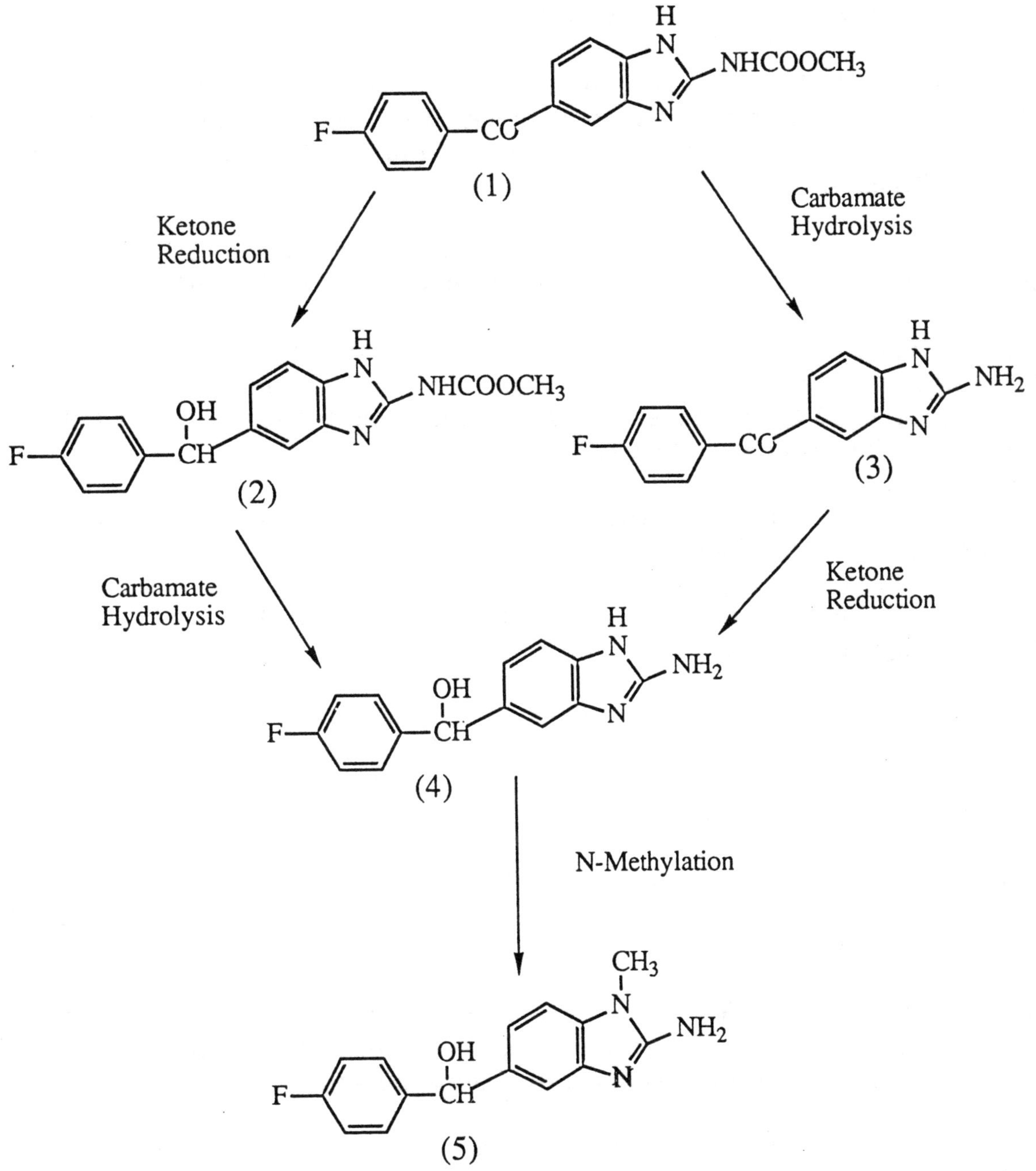

(1) flubendazole
(2) methyl-{5-[α-hydroxy-α-(4-fluorophenyl) methyl]-1H-benzimidazol-2-yl} carbamate (R 38 758)
(3) (2-amino-1H-benzimidazol-5-yl)-4-fluorophenyl-methanone
(4) 2-amino-α-(4-fluorophenyl)-1H-benzimidazole-5-methanol
(5) 2-amino-α-(4-fluorophenyl)-1-methyl-1H-benzimidazole-5-methanol

REFERENCES

Fujisawa Pharmaceutical Co. 1981. Assay of flubendazole by means of high performance liquid chromatography. Unpublished report N 25492. Submitted to FAO by Janssen Pharmaceutica, Beerse, Belgium.

Lee, I.-Y., 1981. Metabolism of flubendazole in swine: Excretion pattern of [2-^{14}C] flubendazole and its metabolites and depletion kinetics of drug residues in edible tissues. Unpublished report V 7902. Submitted to FAO by Janssen Pharmaceutica, Beerse, Belgium.

Marti, A.M., Mooser, A.E., and Koch, H. 1990. Determination of benzimidazole anthelmintics in meat samples. J. Chromatography, 498:145-157.

Meuldermans, W., Hurkmans, R., Swijsen, E., and Heykants, J. 1977. A comparative study on the excretion and metabolism of flubendazole (R 17 889) and mebendazole (R 17 635) in the rat. Unpublished report V 2940. Submitted to FAO by Janssen Pharmaceutica, Beerse, Belgium.

Meuldermans, W., Lee, I.-Y., Hendrickx, J., Swysen, E., Lauwers, W., Porter, D., and Heykants, J. 1982. Metabolism of flubendazole in swine: Excretion pattern of [2-^{14}C] flubendazole and its metabolites and depletion kinetics of drug residues in edible tissues. Unpublished report V 4485. Submitted to FAO by Janssen Pharmaceutica, Beerse, Belgium.

Meuldermans, W., Swijsen, E., Hendrickx, J., Lauwers, W., Bracke, J., Lenaerts, F., Sneyers, R., and Heykants, J. 1978. On the absorption, excretion and biotransformation of flubendazole in the dog. Unpublished report V 2939. Submitted to FAO by Janssen Pharmaceutica, Beerse, Belgium.

Michiels, M., Hendriks, R., Geerts, R., Heykants, J., and Desplenter, L. 1983. Flubendazole residues in eggs and tissues of laying hens. Unpublished report V 4925. Submitted to FAO by Janssen Pharmaceutica, Beerse, Belgium.

Michiels, M., Hendriks, R., Heykants, J., and Marsboom, R. 1979. Residual tissue levels of flubendazole in the pig after a single oral administration. Unpublished report V 3083. Submitted to FAO by Janssen Pharmaceutica, Beerse, Belgium.

Michiels, M., Hendriks, R., Thijssen, J., and Heykants, J. 1978. A sensitive radioimmunoassay for mebendazole (R 17 635) and flubendazole (R 17 889). Unpublished report V 3044. Submitted to FAO by Janssen Pharmaceutica, Beerse, Belgium.

Michiels, M., Heykants, J., and Hendrickx, J. 1977a. Distribution of flubendazole (R 17 889) and its metabolites in the Wistar rat. Unpublished report V 2597. Submitted to FAO by Janssen Pharmaceutica, Beerse, Belgium.

Michiels, M., Heykants, J., Hendrickx, J., Wynants, J., and Marsboom, R. 1976. Residual tissue levels of flubendazole (R 17889) in the pig. Unpublished report V 2483. Submitted to FAO by Janssen Pharmaceutica, Beerse, Belgium.

Michiels, M., Heykants, J., Sneyers, R., Wynants, J., and Marsboom, R. 1977b. Residual tissue levels of flubendazole in the pig after a single oral administration. Unpublished report V 2601. Submitted to FAO by Janssen Pharmaceutica, Beerse, Belgium.

Michiels, M., Heykants, J., Van den Bossche, H., and Verhoeven, H. 1980. A comparative study on the systemic absorption of oral and subcutaneous mebendazole, flubendazole and R 34 803 in two different rodents. Unpublished report N 19702. Submitted to FAO by Janssen Pharmaceutica, Beerse, Belgium.

Tornoe, N., and Christensen, S. undated. Flubendazole residues in hens after treatment with flubendazole medicated food. Unpublished report V 5957. Submitted to FAO by Janssen Pharmaceutica, Beerse, Belgium.

Van Leemput, L., and Heykants, J. 1991. Flubendazole: concentrations in plasma and residues in edible tissues of pheasants after a 7-day treatment at 60 ppm in the feed. Unpublished report number R 17889/FK1071. Submitted to FAO by Janssen Pharmaceutica, Beerse, Belgium.

IVERMECTIN

RESIDUE DEPLETION STUDY

Background

Ivermectin residues, greater than expected after a withdrawal period of 35 days, were observed in livers of heavy cattle (~ 450 kg) treated with ivermectin injectable in New Zealand. The original cattle residue study summarized by the 36th JECFA Meeting was conducted with cattle weighing ~ 260 kg. In view of these new data, a definitive tissue residue study with ivermectin injectable was conducted using cattle weighing 300-400 kg. Cattle in this weight range were considered the most appropriate population in which to assess tissue residue depletion of anthelmintics based upon their use pattern in the cattle industry.

Cattle

Seventy eight crossbred beef cattle aged 12 to 14 months and weighing 297 to 401 kg were used. Seventy two of the animals were given IVOMEC Injection (1% w/v ivermectin) at 1 ml/50 kg, and six animals were used as untreated controls. The allocation of animals is detailed below.

Group	Treatment	Day of Slaughter	Number of Cattle[a]
1	Untreated controls	--[b]	6
2	IVOMEC Injection	21	12
3	IVOMEC Injection	28	12
4	IVOMEC Injection	35	12
5	IVOMEC Injection	42	12
6	IVOMEC Injection	49	12
7	IVOMEC Injection	56	12

[a] Equal number of steers and heifers
[b] One steer and heifer slaughtered on each of days 21, 35 and 56

At slaughter, samples of perirenal fat, both kidneys, the whole liver, skeletal muscle and injection site were collected, homogenized, then measured using HPLC assays developed and validated by the Company. The limit of detection of the assay is 1 ng/g.

Ivermectin (H_2B_{1a}) residue data from tissues of cattle slaughtered on Days 21-49 are summarized below in Table 1. Because tissues at day 49 contained ivermectin residues that were nearly undetectable, tissues from cattle slaughtered on Day 56 post-treatment were not assayed. Ivermectin residues were higher in liver than in fat and lowest in muscle and kidney. On Day 42, all residue values for liver and fat were ≤ 10 ng/g. Ivermectin residues for muscle and kidney were low relative to those of liver and fat and by Day 35 all values for muscle and kidney were near or below the level of detection of the assay. Concentrations of H_2B_{1a} in injection sites of some cattle are ~2500 ng/g at 35 (1/12), 42 (2/12) and 49 (1/12) days post-treatment. Metabolism of ivermectin is not expected in the injection site; therefore, the majority of the total residue is probably parent ivermectin. (Wallace et al., 1992)

Table 1. Concentration (ng/g) of Ivermectin (H_2B_{1a}) in Tissues of Cattle Treated with a Single SC Injection of 0.3 mg/kg

Withdrawal Time (days)	Muscle	Liver	Kidney	Fat	Inj. Site
21	4	46	4	29	NA
28	1	27	2	11	1280
35	1	10	1	6	576
42	0	3	0	2	570
49	0	3	0	1	231

NA - Not assayed

APPRAISAL

JECFA used the residue chemistry data in the monograph developed for the 36th Session of JECFA to recommend MRLs in cattle as follows:

Cattle

Based on the ADI of 0-1 μg/kg established by the 40th JECFA, the permitted maximum daily intake of ivermectin is 60 μg of total drug-related residue contributed by 500 g of food animal meat in the diet of a 60-kg person. At 28 days of withdrawal, the intake of residues of ivermectin is well below the ADI. Based on the data from the metabolism and residue studies, JECFA recommended MRLs of 100 μg/kg for liver and 40 μg/kg for fat (see Table 2).

Table 2. Recommended MRLs for Ivermectin in Cattle

Tissue	Observed Concentration at Day 28 Withdrawal, µg/kg 0.3 mg/kg SC	µg Ivermectin Consumed	µg/kg Recommended MRL (parent)	µg(a) Consumed (Theory)
Muscle	1(1.5)b	0.45	2(3)b	0.9
Liver	27(73)c	7.30	100(270)c	27.0
Kidney	2(3.7)d	0.19	4(7.4)d	1.4
Fat	11(61)e	3.05	40(222)e	11.1
Total		10.99		40.4

a) Based on a daily intake of 0.3 kg muscle, 0.1 kg liver, 0.05 kg kidney and fat.
b) Adjusted observed value by 67% to estimate total residues at 28 days withdrawal.
c) Adjusted observed value by 37% to estimate total residues at 28 days withdrawal.
d) Adjusted observed value by 54% to estimate total residues at 28 days withdrawal.
e) Adjusted observed value by 18% to estimate total residues at 28 days withdrawal.

The concentrations of ivermectin at the injection site were considered significant in regards to their quantity; however, the human toxicological data summarized in the WHO monograph established that the extremely rare consumption of an injection site would not result in an adverse health effect.

REFERENCES

Wallace, D.H., Kunkle, B.N., Maddox, R., Wooden, J.W., Malinski, T.J., Fox, A. and Wehner, T.A. 1992. Unpublished report ASR 13527. Submitted to FAO by Merck, Sharp and Dohme Research Laboratories, Rahway, NJ.

THIABENDAZOLE

IDENTITY

Chemical name: Thiabendazole

CAS Number: 148-79-8

CAS Nomenclature: 2-(4-thiazolyl)-1H-benzimidazole,
4-(2-benzimidazolyl)thiazole

Synonyms: Omnizole, Thiaben, Thibenzole, Bovizole, Eprofil, Equizole, Mintezol, Mertect, Lombristop, Minzolum, Nemapan, Polival, TBZ

Structural formula:

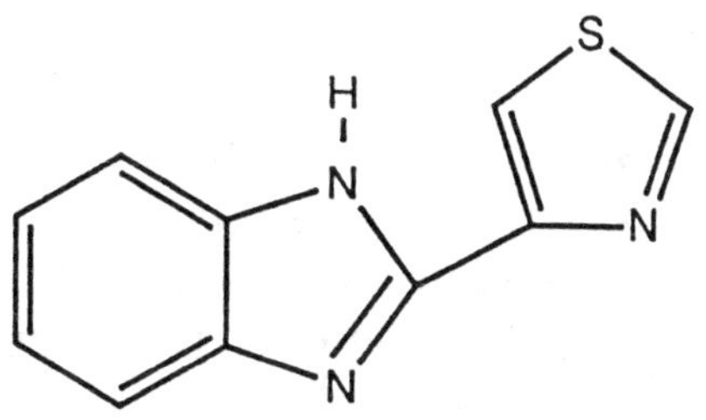

Molecular formula: $C_{10}H_7N_3S$

Molecular weight: 201.3

OTHER INFORMATION ON IDENTITY AND PROPERTIES

Pure active ingredient: Thiabendazole contains not less than 98.0% and not more than 101.0 % $C_{10}H_7N_3S$ calculated on the anhydrous basis. Thiabendazole is a chelating agent and forms stable complexes with a number of metals, including iron. It does not bind calcium.

Appearance: White, crystalline

Melting point: 304-305°C

Solubility: Slightly soluble in water, more soluble in dilute acid and alkali, maximum solubility is at pH 2.2. Soluble in DMF and DMSO.

RESIDUES IN FOOD AND THEIR EVALUATION

CONDITIONS OF USE

General

Thiabendazole is a member of a well-known and widely used chemical class of compounds known as the benzimidazoles. It is related in chemical structure and pharmacological properties to other compounds such as fenbendazole, oxibendazole, oxfendazole, mebendazole, febantel and triclabendazole.

Thiabendazole is a potent, orally effective, broad spectrum anthelmintic with significant activity against gastrointestinal parasites in cattle, swine, sheep, goats, poultry, horses, dogs and many species of exotic animals. In addition, thiabendazole has been found to be effective in the control of a large number of fungal diseases affecting plants, animals and man.

Dosages

Thiabendazole is administered orally to cattle (3-5 g/100 lb BW), sheep (2 g/100 lb BW), and goats (2-3 g/100 lb BW) as a suspension, medicated feed, bolus, drench or as top dressing pellets. Additionally, it is available for cattle as an oral paste (3-5 g/100 lb BW) and in a medicated block (0.33 lb of block/100 lb BW). Preparations available for swine include an oral paste (30-40 mg/lb BW) and a premix (0.05-0.1% thiabendazole/ton feed).

METABOLISM

General

Metabolic studies have shown that thiabendazole is rapidly absorbed, metabolized, and excreted in man, cattle, rats, sheep, dogs, and goats. Excretion generally is completed within 3 to 8 days via urine and feces. In cows, approximately 0.1% of the dose was excreted in milk within 60 hours. The major metabolite found in all species studied was 5-hydroxythiabendazole, as a glucuronide or sulfate ester.

Rat

Eight rats were given single oral doses of ^{14}C or ^{35}S labeled thiabendazole and blood, urine, and feces samples were radiometrically analyzed (Tocco 1966). In 4 rats dosed with 100 mg/kg, maximum concentrations of drug and metabolites in whole blood were found 2 to 6 hours after dosing and ranged from 15 to 24 μg/ml. In 4 rats dosed with 25 mg/kg, 92% of the dose was excreted with 66% in urine and 26% in feces by 48 hours post treatment. After the 100 mg/kg dose, 79% of the dose was excreted by 48 hours with 49% in urine and 30% in feces. After 48 hours through day 8, excretion was close to the limit of detection at 0.1 μg/ml. Using paper chromatography, the composition of 24 hour urine from one rat dosed with 25 mg/kg was identified as unchanged thiabendazole (3%), free 5-hydroxythiabendazole (4%), the sulfate conjugate of 5-hydroxythiabendazole (39%), and the glucuronide conjugate of 5-hydroxythiabendazole (50%).

Radioactivity was not detected in the carcass of rats dosed with 25 mg/kg and sacrificed after 14 days.

Dog

Four dogs, given a single oral dose of 50 mg/kg body weight of thiabendazole-^{14}C, had urine, feces, and plasma analyzed radiometrically and spectrofluorometrically (Tocco 1966). Metabolites appeared in the plasma 30 minutes after dosing and reached maximum levels of 7 to 21 µg/ml within 2 hours. Three days after dosing, an average of 82% of thiabendazole was excreted, with 35% in urine and 47% in feces.

Cattle

Eighteen calves were administered single oral doses of 50 to 200 mg/kg thiabendazole (^{14}C, ^{3}H, or nonradioactive) in capsules or in a drench suspension. Urine, blood, feces samples were analyzed radiometrically and spectrofluorometrically. In results reported for 3 calves dosed with 50 and 200 mg/kg, plasma concentrations peaked from 4 to 7 hours (Tocco 1965; Anonymous 1981). In 2 calves dosed with 50 mg/kg, plasma concentrations were zero by 2 days. In one calf dosed with 200 mg/kg, the plasma concentration was 0.3 µg/ml on day 8, the last day of collection. In results reported for 4 calves (3 dosed with 50 mg/kg and one dosed with 200 mg/kg), 63% of the drug was excreted after 4 days with 55% in the urine and 8% (determined spectrofluorometrically) or 30% (determined radiometrically) in the feces (Tocco 1965; Anonymous 1981). After a 50 mg/kg dose, radioactivity was undetectable in urine by day 10 (Tocco 1965). By 40 days, radioactivity was undetectable in urine after a dose of 150 mg/kg. It took 45 to 50 days for radioactivity in urine to drop to undetectable levels after a dose of 200 mg/kg. In 3 animals, after the 50 mg/kg dose, tissue residues determined by spectrofluorometry were barely detectable (detection limit = 0.2 µg/g wet tissue), 3 days after treatment and in 1 calf radioactivity was not detected in tissue after 30 days (Tocco 1965). In 12 animals, after a 110 mg/kg dose, residues were not detected 3, 7, and 14 days after dosing (Anonymous 1981). In one calf, 57 days after 200 mg/kg dose, all tissue residues were at or below 0.6 ppm and 4 tissues had levels below the detection limit of the radiometric method (0.07 ppm) (Tocco 1965). In another calf, 34 days after the 110 mg/kg dose, radioactivity levels were highest in liver at 1.5 µg/g by radiometric analysis (Tocco 1965). Spectrofluorometric analysis did not agree with radiometric results in 2 cases. This discrepancy may be due to degradation of labeled thiabendazole.

Eight dairy cows were given 3, 5, or 10 g/100 lbs thiabendazole drench formulation or 5 g/100 lbs thiabendazole bolus formulation (Tocco 1965). Recovery of thiabendazole and metabolites ranged from 72 to 120% for compounds with concentrations between 0.05 to 5.0 ppm. Approximately 0.1% of the dose was excreted in milk with over 99% of the drug present as metabolites. Highest concentrations of thiabendazole and metabolites appeared within 24 hours after dosing. Residues were not detected 60 hours after dosing.

The absorption and pharmacokinetics of fenbendazole and thiabendazole in cattle were compared (Prichard *et al.* 1981). Three cattle were dosed intraruminally with

5 mg fenbendazole/kg, 100 mg thiabendazole/kg and the marker, chromium ethylenediaminetetraacetate (Cr-EDTA). Samples of digesta, blood, urine and feces were analyzed by spectrofluorometry. Drug movement through the gastrointestinal tract was derived by compartmental analysis of Cr-EDTA concentrations and integration of benzimidazole concentrations. Approximately 12% of thiabendazole left the rumen in digesta, indicating a net absorption from the rumen of 88%. No metabolites of thiabendazole were found in rumen contents. Elimination of thiabendazole from the rumen was virtually complete within 48 hours of administration. Approximately 10% and 8% of the thiabendazole dose appeared at the pylorus and terminal ileum, respectively. Of these amounts, 9% in the abomasum and practically 100% in the ileum was present as 5-hydroxythiabendazole, indicating that metabolites of absorbed thiabendazole were recycled to the GI tract. Thiabendazole reached maximum levels (about 3 mg/L) in plasma approximately 4 hours after treatment. Thiabendazole plasma levels dropped to about 0.3 mg/L at 24 hours. At 0.5 hours, 5-hydroxythiabendazole was present and contributed about half of the total thiabendazole in plasma throughout sampling. Between 17 and 36% of thiabendazole dose was excreted in the first 24 hour urine with urinary thiabendazole excretion ceasing 40 hours after dosing. Approximately 5% of the total urinary excretion occurred as unchanged drug.

The plasma concentrations of anthelmintics and their metabolites were compared (Prichard *et al. 1985*). Ten cattle were treated with fenbendazole, oxfendazole, febantel, albendazole, and thiabendazole using seven treatment procedures. Three cattle were treated with 176 g/L (from 88 mg/kg concentration) by oral drench. Plasma samples were analyzed by HPLC with a limit of detection of 70 ng/ml. The parent compound was not detected. The levels of 5-hydroxythiabendazole peaked at approximately 2 µg/ml by 4 hours post treatment. By 30 hours post dosing, the levels of 5-hydroxythiabendazole dropped to approximately 0.1 µg/ml.

<u>Swine</u>

Eleven young pigs were dosed with thiabendazole (nonradioactive, ^{14}C, ^{3}H, or ^{35}S) by feed or by capsule. During the medicated feeding of 0.02% feed for 4 days, plasma levels of thiabendazole in 2 pigs ranged from 1.2 to 2.0 µg/ml and were undetectable in 30 days (Anonymous 1981). The limit of detection was 0.02 ppm for thiabendazole and 0.05 ppm for total 5-hydroxythiabendazole. In 4 pigs dosed 50 mg/kg, an average of 76% of the drug was excreted with 66% in urine and 10% in feces in 3 days (Tocco 1965). Only 2 pigs out of 11 had significant drug radioactivity in tissues. One pig treated with a single dose of 50 mg/kg had the highest residue value in large intestine (0.36 µg/g) at 10 days withdrawal (Tocco 1965). The second pig after being treated with 0.02% feed for 4 days had the highest residue value in liver (8.9 µg/ml) at 1 day withdrawal (Anonymous 1981). Questionable or invalid data was reported for some plasma and tissue samples. It was suggested that accidental contamination of samples occurred during analysis. Eight pigs dosed with 0.1% nonradioactive thiabendazole feed for 17 days, and then fed 0.02% for 4 weeks with 30 day withdrawal had an average residue of 0.08 ppm in liver and 0.40 ppm in kidney determined by spectrofluorometric method; no residues were found in muscle (Anonymous 1981).

Sheep

Twenty-two sheep orally received 50, 100, or 200 mg/kg thiabendazole (nonradioactive, ^{14}C, or ^{35}S). Plasma, tissue, urine and feces samples were analyzed radiometrically and spectrofluorometrically. After 50 mg/kg dose, plasma concentrations of thiabendazole in 5 sheep peaked between 4 and 8 hours after dosing with values ranging from 7.7 to 10.4 μg/ml (Anonymous 1981). In 4 days after a 50 mg/kg dose, 8 sheep excreted an average of 89% of the drug, 75% in urine and 14% in feces (Tocco *et al.* 1964). Tissue residues of radioactivity in one sheep which received 50 mg/kg thiabendazole were highest in cecum (34.4 mg/g), small intestine (33.6 mg/g) and kidney (13.9 μg/g) at 6 hours after dosing (Tocco *et al.* 1964). At five days post treatment, residues were low and by 24 days, residues were below detection (0.06 μg/g). Tissue residues of radioactivity in 2 sheep that received 100 mg/kg were highest in bladder (average 0.26), spleen (average 0.26), skin (0.38 and 0.44), and pancreas (0.66, 0.08) (Anonymous 1981). With 1 day withdrawal, twelve sheep dosed orally with 100 and 200 mg nonradioactive thiabendazole/kg had the following residues: muscle - 0.36 to 3.87, liver - 2.05 to 3.69, kidney - 1.11 to 3.80. At 7 and 28 days after treatment, residues were below the detection limit of 0.2 μg/g (Anonymous 1981).

Goat

Seven goats were orally treated with 50 or 150 mg/kg thiabendazole (^{3}H, or ^{35}S and ^{14}C) (Tocco *et al.* 1965). Plasma, tissue, urine and feces samples were analyzed radiometrically and spectrofluorometrically. After 50 or 150 mg/kg dose, plasma concentrations of thiabendazole from 7 goats peaked between 2 and 8 hours with values ranging from 1.9 to 10.9 μg/ml (Tocco *et al.* 1965; Anonymous 1981). After 24 hours, plasma levels dropped substantially. At time of sacrifice (from 1 to 30 days), 6 goats dosed with 50 or 150 mg/kg excreted an average of 85% of the drug with 59% in urine and 26% in feces (Tocco *et al.* 1965). In tissue of goats that received thiabendazole, highest levels of residues appeared in abomasum (2.1 μg/g), kidney (2.7 μg/g) and large intestine (2.3 μg/g) after 24 hours. By 17 days post dosing, residue levels were zero except in abomasum (0.25 μg/g), heart (0.2 μg/g), large intestine (0.35 μg/g), liver (0.2 μg/g), and lung (0.1 μg/g). By 30 days post dosing, all residues were zero. In six goats given a thiabendazole drench formulation in dosages of 50, 150, or 225 mg/kg, approximately 1% of the dose was secreted in milk with the highest levels of thiabendazole and metabolites appeared within 24 hours (Tocco *et al.* 1965). Ninety percent of the drug was present as metabolites. No drug or metabolites were detectable in the milk 4 days later.

Man

Four male subjects were dosed with a suspension of 1.0 g ^{14}C-thiabendazole (Tocco *et al.* 1966). Plasma drug concentrations were measured radiometrically (detection level 0.2 ppm) and spectrofluorometrically (detection level 0.1 ppm for thiabendazole and 0.2 ppm for its metabolites). Plasma concentrations of thiabendazole peaked from 1-2 hours after treatment with values ranging from 13 to 18 μg/ml and then dropping to the detection level between 24 and 48 hours.

By 48 hours, 87 to 100% of the dose was excreted in the urine (81-91%) and feces (2-7%). Twenty-five percent of the dose detected in the urine was glucuronide and 13% was sulfate esters of 5-hydroxythiabendazole. Less than 1% of the dose was excreted as unchanged thiabendazole or unconjugated 5-hydroxythiabendazole. After 5 days, 4 to 9% of the dose was excreted in feces.

Twelve male subjects were dosed with 2 g thiabendazole in the form of tablets, wafers, capsules, and suspension in a cross-over experiment (Anonymous 1981). Plasma concentrations of thiabendazole peaked about 3 hours after treatment with values ranging from 11 to 18 μg/ml. Thiabendazole in the wafer was more rapidly absorbed with peak values of 30 to 50% higher than the other forms. For all 4 forms, sixteen to 21% of the drug was excreted in the urine after 24 hours.

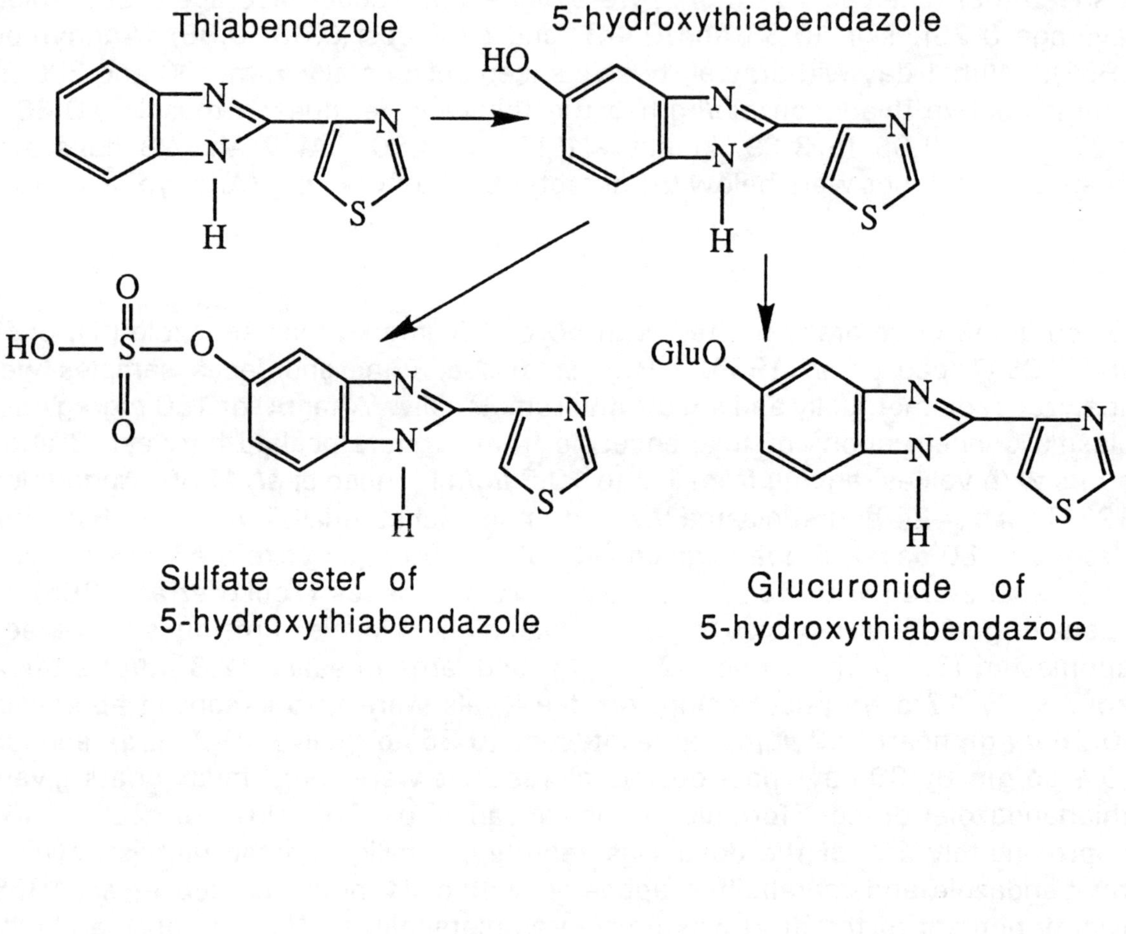

TISSUE RESIDUE DEPLETION STUDIES

Radiolabeled Residue Depletion Studies

Rat

In a series of studies, rats were divided into four treatment groups. Rats were treated with ^{14}C-thiabendazole, alone or with sodium formate, with $NaH^{14}CO_3$ and with $H^{14}COONa$. Total excretion of thiabendazole was 69-99% in rats receiving ^{14}C-thiabendazole alone and 96-97% for rats receiving ^{14}C-thiabendazole with sodium formate. Terminal excretion rates and tissue retention of radioactivity were similar for all three compounds. Table 1 shows the residues in tissues of rats treated with ^{14}C-thiabendazole, $NaH^{14}CO_3$ and $H^{14}COONa$ (Anonymous 1981).

Table 1. Tissue residues (μg/g) in the Rat

Compound	Dose (mg/kg)	Kidney	Liver	Carcass	Terminal Excretion (Days $^{-1}$)
^{14}C-Thiabendazole	96	0.04	DL	0.19	-0.032
	173	0.07	0.03	0.46	-0.031
^{14}C-Thiabendazole + Formate	110	0.02	DL	0.10	-0.040
	202	0.04	0.02	0.13	-0.042
$NaH^{14}CO_3$	1.7	0.00047	0.00034	0.00013	-0.017
	2280	0.53	0.62	1.5	-0.016
$H^{14}COONa$	20.3	0.096	0.053	0.34	-0.033
	4570	3.26	2.74	8.5	-0.028

DL = Detection Limits

The study suggests that all three compounds contribute to a common carbon pool of small molecules that are subsequently incorporated into other molecules. Radioactive residues resulting from administration of ^{14}C-thiabendazole would, by extension, be the products of reincorporation from this common carbon pool and not a measure of thiabendazole residues.

Cattle

A single calf was treated orally with a capsule containing ^{3}H-thiabendazole at a dose of 50 mg/kg. Ninety percent of the administered dose was recovered in the urine and feces (65% and 25%, respectively). Plasma drug concentrations are shown in Table 2. At a detection limit of 0.08 ppm there were no detectable tissue residues 30 days following treatment.

Table 2. Concentration (μg/ml) of thiabendazole in the plasma of a calf treated with 50 mg/kg ^{3}H-Thiabendazole

Time after Dosing (h)	Concentration (μg/ml)
1	0.5
2	0.8
4	1.8
6	2.0
7	NA
24	≤1

Three calves were treated orally via capsule with ^{14}C-thiabendazole at doses of 110, 150 and 200 mg/kg. Calves were slaughtered 34, 59 and 57 days postdosing. At the 200 mg/kg dose, 81% of the administered dose was excreted in the urine and feces (47 % and 34 %, respectively). Plasma drug concentrations are shown in Table 3. Tissue residues at slaughter are shown in Table 4 (Anonymous 1981).

Table 3. Concentration (μg/ml) of thiabendazole in the plasma a calf treated orally with 200 mg/kg ^{14}C-Thiabendazole

Time after Dosing	Concentration (μg/ml)
1 h	4.1
2	5.0
4	7.5
6	NA
7	9.6
24	3.8
2 days	1.3
3	1.1
4	0.4
5	0.5
6	0.5
7	0.4
8	0.3

Table 4. Tissue residues (ppm) in calves treated orally with ^{14}C-Thiabendazole

Tissue	Dose (mg/kg) [Sacrifice, days]		
	110 [34]	150 [59]	200 [57]
Fat	0.1*	0.0**	0.18*
Kidney	0.15	0.11	0.13
Liver	1.5	0.39	0.59
Muscle	0	0.13	0.16

* Estimated detection limit ≈ 0.08
**Estimated detection limit ≈ 0.07

As simultaneous determination of thiabendazole residues using spectrofluorometric analysis showed only very low residues, a series of fractionation studies were conducted to demonstrate that the radioactivity measured in the tissues of treated calves was the result of the degradation of labeled thiabendazole and subsequent incorporation of small molecules containing ^{14}C into several metabolic cycles (Anonymous 1981).

Fractionation of liver from a calf treated with 200 mg/kg ^{14}C-Thiabendazole:

Procedure 1 utilizes a methylene chloride extraction of the acid hydrolyzate of ^{14}C-thiabendazole-containing liver. At a detection limit of 0.16 μg thiabendazole (of the ≈12 μg/20 g tissue sample), negligible residues, indistinguishable from the control, were detected. The method accounts for approximately 1% of the anticipated residue.

Procedure 2 also employs an initial methylene chloride extraction. The aqueous phase that results is extracted with ethyl acetate and back extracted with 0.1 N HCl. The majority of the radiolabel is detected in the solid residue following combustion analysis. The method accounts for approximately 60% of the anticipated residue.

Procedure 3 utilizes an acid hydrolysis followed by chromatography on resin. The acid eluate accounts for approximately 4% of the expected residue. The major fractions are the basic eluate (49%), containing the bulk of the amino acids, and the solid residue (39%, after combustion analysis). No residue is associated with the spent resin. Accountability is approximately 90%.

Procedure 4 uses salt extraction at pH 5.5 and pH 10.0. Approximately 60% of the activity is in the acidic fraction. An additional 18% is found in the basic fraction. Solid residues contain approximately 20% of the residues.

Procedures 6 and 7 produce purified nucleic acid and protein fractions. Recoveries range from 65% for nucleic acids to 90% for proteins. Radioactivity in the nucleic acid fraction is negligible. The protein fraction contains approximately 25% of the anticipated thiabendazole.

Fractionation of liver from a calf treated with 110 mg/kg ^{14}C-Thiabendazole:

Procedure 4 demonstrated an accountability of approximately 90%. Radioactivity is extracted at both pH 5.5 (29%) and pH 10.0 (36%). Approximately 25 % remains in the solid material.

Procedure 5 results in the separation and identification of lipid and polysaccharide fractions from the liver tissue. Radioactivity is essentially absent from those fractions anticipated to contain thiabendazole or its metabolite. The lipid fraction contains approximately 14% of the initial radioactivity and the polysaccharide fraction contains ≈ 1%. Upon combustion, the solid residue contains 34% of the expected radioactivity. The polysaccharide filtrate, containing protein hydrolysate and other water soluble constituents, contains ≈ 29% of the radioactivity. Accountability is approximately 80%.

Procedure 7 results in isolation of protein from the liver tissue. Protein contains approximately 60% of the initial radioactivity. Nonprecipitating material accounts for approximately 14% of the total and 12% is attributed to fatty material. Total accountability is approximately 85%.

From procedures 5 and 7 the company concludes that the radioactivity is not restricted to a single component or fraction. The "residues" derived from calves treated with radiolabeled thiabendazole are apparent rather than real.

<u>Sheep</u>

Two lambs were treated orally with 50 mg/kg ^{14}C-thiabendazole. Total urine and feces were analyzed. Table 5 shows the percent of the dose excreted in 96 hours (Tocco 1960).

Table 5. Urinary and fecal excretion (% of total) of ^{14}C-thiabendazole following an oral dose of 50 mg/kg in lambs

	Time After Dose (h)	Lamb No 981	Lamb No 979
Urine	96	77	74
Feces	96	14	16

OTHER RESIDUE DEPLETION STUDIES

Cattle

Fifteen calves were treated with thiabendazole via capsule (950 mg/kg) or drench (50 or 110 mg/kg). Plasma levels of drug were determined in one calf and tissue residues were analyzed in three animals treated at 50 mg/kg and slaughtered at one and three days postdosing. A fluorometric assay was used (detection limit of 0.2 µg/g). Tissue residues were low at one day postdosing, negligible to absent after three days, and absent in samples collected more than three days after drug treatment (Anonymous 1981)

Two Friesian cows in midlactation were given thiabendazole orally, at a dose of 66 mg/kg. Cows were milked twice daily at approximately 12 hour intervals. Milk samples were collected at 12, 24, 36, 48, 60, 72, 84, 96, 108, 120, 132 and 144 hours after treatment. Milk was analyzed for thiabendazole residues as whole milk and, following fractionation into aqueous (whey) and lipid (curds) phases, the aqueous phase was analyzed. With an assay limit of detection of 0.5 µg/ml, neither thiabendazole nor its 5-OH metabolite were detected in any of the samples (Weir 1987).

Table 6. Residues (µg/ml) of thiabendazole and its 5-OH metabolite in milk

Sample	Dose (g/100 lbs)	Formulation	TBZ	5-OH-TBZ
0-12	3	drench	0.06	2.39
12-24			ND	1.10
24-36			ND	0.26
36-48			ND	0.07
48-60			ND	0.02
60-72			ND	ND
0-12	5	drench	0.03	3.59
12-24			0.03	2.08
24-36			ND	0.79
36-48			ND	0.15
48-60			ND	0.05
60-72			ND	ND
0-12	10	drench	0.22	4.14
12-24			0.05	3.82
24-36			ND	0.83
36-48			ND	0.29
48-60			ND	0.09
60-72			ND	ND
0-12	5	bolus	0.16	3.27
12-24			ND	2.15
24-36			ND	0.53
36-48			ND	0.17
48-60			ND	0.03
60-72			ND	ND

Six dairy cows were treated orally via drench with thiabendazole at doses of 3, 5 or 10 g/100 lbs. Two other cows were given thiabendazole in a bolus formulation at a dose of 5 g/100 lbs. The animals were milked at 12 hour intervals for six days. Milk was analyzed for thiabendazole and its 5-OH metabolite (including 5-glucuronide and 5-OSO_3). Samples were analyzed spectrofluorometrically. The assay has a limit of quantitation of 0.05 μg/ml. Residues of thiabendazole and its 5-OH metabolites are shown in Table 6 (Robinson et al. 1963).

Seven Friesian cows were divided into control and treatment groups. Control animals received an oral drench with water equivalent in volume to the largest volume given to cows in the treatment group. Animals in the treatment group received a 17.6% preformed suspension of thiabendazole at a dose of 66 mg/kg. Milk samples were collected prior to treatment and at 8, 24, 32, 48, 72 and 108 hours after dosing. High pressure liquid chromatography with fluorescence detection was used to measure the concentration of thiabendazole residues in the milk. Results of the study are shown in Table 7 (Batty et al. 1985).

Table 7. Mean residues (ppm) of thiabendazole and 5-OH thiabendazole in the milk of treated cows

Sample	TBZ	5-OH-TBZ	Total
0	0	0	0
8	<0.1*	0.93	0.97
24	<0.1	1.05	1.07
32	<0.1	<0.1	<0.1
48	<0.1	<0.1	<0.1

* Limit of detection = 0.1 ppm

Nine lactating Holstein cows were treated orally with encapsulated thiabendazole at doses of 0.5, 1.5 and 5.0 g daily for a period of 28 days. Two control animals received cellulose-filled gelatin capsules. Two cows from each treatment group were slaughtered at the end of the 28-day treatment period. One control cow was euthanized on day 14 of the treatment period due to poor health. At the end of the 28 day dosing period (study day 29), all cows but one from each treatment group were humanly killed to obtain tissues for residues analysis. The remaining cows were slaughtered after a 28-day washout period. Milk samples were collected on days -1, 1, 2, 4, 7, 14, 21, 28, 29, 35, 42 and 56. Subsamples of 500 ml were composited on each sample day and retained for analysis. Tissues were collected for residue analysis at the time of slaughter. Residues were determined spectrofluorometrically. Summaries of milk residues are shown in Tables 8 and 9. A summary of tissue residues are shown in Table 10 (Predmore and Justin 1987).

Table 8. Summary of milk residues (Days 2 - 28)[ppm]

		TBZ		5-OH-TBZ		Total†	
Dose	Cow No	Range	Mean	Range	Mean	Range	Mean
Control*	8	0.010-0.019	0.014	0.001-0.005	0.003	0.013-0.024	0.017
0.5	14	0.010-0.018	0.014	0.010-0.012	0.010	0.020-0.028	0.024
	22	0.014-0.017	0.016	0.016-0.018	0.017	0.030-0.036	0.033
	9	0.010-0.014	0.012	0.010-0.013	0.010	0.020-0.025	0.022
1.5	7	0.010-0.014	0.013	0.116-0.148	0.135	0.130-0.162	0.148
	10	0.014-0.018	0.016	0.016-0.096	0.042	0.033-0.112	0.058
	12	0.012-0.016	0.014	0.082-0.091	0.087	0.098-0.105	0.101
5.0	3	0.011-0.022	0.016	0.143-0.2446	0.176	0.159-0.262	0.192
	6	0.014-0.018	0.016	0.064-0.092	0.081	0.082-0.106	0.097
	15	0.014-0.016	0.015	0.090-0.103	0.096	0.105-0.123	0.112

* Data from the entire study period days -1 - day 57
† Total = TBZ + 5-OH-TBZ

Table 9. Summary of milk residues (Days 35 - 56)[ppm]

		TBZ		5-OH-TBZ		Total†	
Dose	Cow No	Range	Mean	Range	Mean	Range	Mean
Control	8	0.014-0.016	0.015	0.002-0.004	0.003	0.017-0.019	0.018
0.5	22	0.010-0.015	0.013	0.002-0.004	0.003	0.012-0.019	0.016
1.5	7	0.013-0.014	0.014	0.004-0.006	0.005	0.017-0.020	0.018
5.0	15	0.012-0.018	0.016	0.002-0.004	0.003	0.016-0.020	0.018

† Total = TBZ + 5-OH-TBZ

Table 10. Summary of mean tissue residues (ppm)

Tissue	Dose	TBZ		5-OH-TBZ		Total	
		Day 29	Day 57	Day 29	Day 57	Day 29	Day 57
Blood	Control	0.014	0.013	0.002	0.004	0.016	0.017
	0.5	0.015	0.013	0.004	0.004	0.019	0.017
	1.5	0.013	0.012	0.015	0.003	0.028	0.015
	5.0	0.016	0.013	0.019	0.004	0.035	0.017
Fat	Control	0.017	0.016	0.002	0.003	0.019	0.019
	0.5	0.017	0.016	0.003	0.003	0.020	0.019
	1.5	0.015	0.016	0.010	0.002	0.025	0.018
	5.0	0.015	0.017	0.009	0.002	0.024	0.019
Kidney	Control	0.018	0.021	0.009	0.010	0.027	0.031
	0.5	0.012	0.020	0.044	0.010	0.056	0.030
	1.5	0.016	0.020	0.25*	0.008	0.27*	0.028
	5.0	0.027	0.022	0.439	0.014	0.466	0.036
Liver	Control	0.016	0.021	0.012	0.020	0.028	0.041
	0.5	0.022	0.018	0.027	0.016	0.049	0.034
	1.5	0.048	0.018	0.086	0.015	0.134	0.033
	5.0	0.068	0.020	0.138	0.017	0.206	0.037
Muscle	Control	0.015	0.013	0.003	0.002	0.018	0.015
	0.5	0.013	0.014	0.002	0.000	0.015	0.014
	1.5	0.014	0.012	0.005	0.002	0.019	0.014
	5.0	0.016	0.016	0.005	0.002	0.021	0.016

* Report offers no explanation for these anomolously high residue values.

Sheep

Three sheep were dosed orally with thiabendazole. One animal was treated at a rate of 60 mg/kg and slaughtered four hours after dosing. Two animals were slaughtered seven days after being treated with either 82 mg/kg or 100 mg/kg. Concentrations of thiabendazole in the plasma and erythrocytes were determined in the sheep receiving the 82 mg/kg dose and are shown in Table 11 (Tocco 1960). Tissue residues resulting from this study are shown in Table 12.

Table 11. Concentration of thiabendazole in the plasma and erythrocytes of a sheep treated orally with 82 mg thiabendazole/kg

Time after dose (h)	Conc. in Plasma (µg/ml)	Conc. in Erythrocytes (µg/ml)
1	0.06	0.08
2	0.28	0.29
3	0.53	0.54
4	1.51	1.54
5	1.00	1.39
6	1.06	1.22
24	0.01	0.01

Thiabendazole concentration in the blood at 24 hours postdosing are consistent with control levels in the blood of untreated sheep.

Table 12. Tissue residues (µg/g) of thiabendazole in sheep

	Dose [Slaughter]		
Tissue	60 mg/kg [4 h]	82 mg/kg [7 days]	100 mg/kg [7 days]
Muscle	0.38	0.02	0.02
Kidney	0.68	0.03	0.03
Liver	4.12	0.04	0.09
Heart Fat	4.40	NA	0.04
Omental Fat	NA	NA	0.03

Tissue residues of thiabendazole were low, even at four hours postdosing when blood levels appeared to be maximal. Recoveries based on internal standards were greater than 90%.

Only 4% of the administered dose was recovered in urine and feces. Two metabolites were detected and were under investigation (Tocco 1960).

Fourteen sheep were maintained on a continuous diet containing various amounts of thiabendazole (TBZ). Blood levels were determined in the treated sheep and in four untreated controls. Results are shown in Table 13 (Tocco 1960).

Table 13. Concentration of thiabendazole in the blood of sheep maintained on a continuous diet of TBZ in feed

TBZ in Feed (%)	Wethers		Females	
	No. of Sheep	Conc. (μg/ml)	No. of Sheep	Conc. (μg/ml)
None	2	0.01*	2	0.03*
0.01	1	0.00	2	0.00
0.032	1	0.01	2	0.01
0.1	2	0.04	2	0.03
0.32	1	0.09	2	0.52
1.0	1	0.47	NA	NA

* Control values have been subtracted from experimental blood sample values

Four sheep were treated orally with thiabendazole at a dose of 44 mg/kg. Animals were slaughtered 1, 2, 3 and 4 days postdosing. Both thiabendazole and its 5-OH metabolite were measured in the tissues. The results are shown in Table 14 (Weir 1987).

Table 14. **Residues (μg/g) of thiabendazole and its 5-OH metabolite in the tissues of sheep treated orally with 44 mg thiabendazole/kg**

Tissue	Withdrawal (days)	Animal No.	TBZ	5-OH-TBZ
Liver	1	91	2.24	2.44
	2	92	0.31	ND
	3	93	0.80	ND
	4	94	ND	ND
Muscle	1	91	0.34	0.24
	2	92	ND	ND
	3	93	ND	ND
	4	94	ND	ND

ND = Not detectable (limit of detection = 0.05 μg/g)

Six Finn-Dorset crossbred lambs were given thiabendazole orally at a dose of 44 mg/kg. Blood samples were collected before drug administration and at 2, 4, 6, 8, 12, 24, 36, 48 and 72 hours after treatment. Samples were assayed for thiabendazole and its 5-OH metabolite. Maximum blood concentrations of thiabendazole were detected between two and four hours postdosing. Measurable levels of thiabendazole were still present at 24 hours postadministration but were absent in the 36 hour collections. The 5-OH metabolite was present in the plasma, reaching a maximum concentration at six hours postdosing. Detectable levels of metabolite were present in the 12 hour samples but concentrations were below the limit of detection by 24 hours. Mean concentrations of thiabendazole and 5-OH-thiabendazole are shown in Table 15 (Weir 1987).

Table 15. **Mean plasma concentrations of thiabendazole and 5-OH-thiabendazole in sheep given thiabendazole orally at a dose of 44 mg/kg**

Time (h)	Thiabendazole (μg/ml)	5-OH-Thiabendazole (μg/ml)
0	0	0
2	2.01 ± 0.87	0.13 ± 0.04
4	2.16 ± 0.88	0.16 ± 0.05
6	1.66 ± 0.77	0.18 ± 0.07
8	1.38 ± 0.70	0.16 ± 0.04
12	0.27 ± 0.23	0.13 ± 0.08
24	0.02 ± 0.01	ND
36	ND	ND
48	ND	ND
72	ND	ND

Concentrations of thiabendazole are higher and persist longer in liver than residues in muscle or plasma (Weir and Bogan 1985).

<u>Swine</u>

Eight crossbred swine were given a single oral dose of 100 mg thiabendazole/kg. The dose was administered as a drench suspension. Pigs were given free access to water and were fed a nonmedicated hog feed. Four pigs were slaughtered seven days after dosing and four pigs were slaughtered 28 days after dosing. Four untreated controls were also slaughtered at the later time. Tissues were assayed for thiabendazole and metabolites using a spectrofluorometric method. The detection sensitivity for the method is 0.05 ppm thiabendazole + metabolites. Assay values for the control swine were at or below the detection limit. The assay values for the treated swine at both 7 and 28 days postdosing were also below the limit of detection (Anonymous 1981).

Three pigs were maintained for two weeks on a diet containing 0.1% thiabendazole. The pigs were slaughtered at zero, 2 and 7 days withdrawal from medicated feed. Tissues were analyzed for thiabendazole and the 5-glucuronide and 5-OSO_3 metabolites. Results for selected tissues are shown in Table 16 (Anonymous 1981).

Table 16. Tissue residues (μg/g) of thiabendazole and its 5-glucuronide and 5-OSO_3 metabolites in pigs receiving 0.1% TBZ in feed for 2 weeks

	Liver			Kidney			Muscle			Fat		
	TBZ	5-OH	Total	TBZ	5-OH	Total	TBZ	5-OH	Total	TBZ	5-OH	Total
Control*	0.02	0.09	0.11	0.03	0.09	0.12	0.04	0.04	0.08	0.05	0.04	0.09
0	3.9	1.8	5.7	2.7	5.3	8.0	2.1	0.16	2.3	3.5	0.22	3.7
2	0.12	0	0.12	0.19	0	0.19	0	0	0	0.17	0	0.17
7	0.05	0	0.05	0	0	0	0	0	0	0.02	0	0.02

*Control values have been subtracted from experimental tissue sample values

METHODS OF ANALYSIS FOR RESIDUES IN TISSUES

A radiometric method was used for thiabendazole, labeled with ^{3}H, or ^{35}S and ^{14}C, in urine, plasma and tissue samples and analyzed by liquid scintillation and low beta Geiger counting (Tocco *et al.* 1965). Feces samples were analyzed by gas proportional counting. The detection limit for tissue was 0.08 μg/g.

A chemical method first extracted thiabendazole and 5-hydroxythiabendazole into ethyl acetate and then into hydrochloric acid for urine, tissue, plasma, and milk samples (Tocco *et al.* 1965). In liver and kidney samples, the glucuronide and sulfate esters of 5-hydroxythiabendazole were first converted to 5-hydroxythiabendazole using β-glucuronidase and sulfatase (glusulase - commercial enzyme mixture), and then extracted. Feces were first extracted with methylene chloride and then hydrochloric acid. Fluorescence was measured by a spectrofluorometer. Thiabendazole and 5-hydroxythiabendazole were recovered with adequate precision (95 $\pm$ 6%) for values from 0.1 to 5 μg/g for plasma and tissue and from 5 to 10 μg/g for urine and feces. The detection limit for tissue was 0.1 μg/g for thiabendazole and 0.2 μg/g for its metabolites. The detection limit for milk was 0.05 μg/g.

A high-performance liquid chromatographic method for measuring eight benzimidazoles in liver, kidney, and muscle was reported (Marti *et al.* 1990). Tissue samples were homogenized with acetonitrile and defatted with hexane. Sodium chloride was added and three phases formed. The hexane layer was discarded, and the remaining two layers were mixed with dichloromethane. The acetonitrile layer was dried over sodium sulfate and evaporated first in a rotovap, then in an N-Evap. The extract was cleaned by passage through a Sep-Pak C_{18} cartridge, evaporated to 0.2 ml and cleaned by a Sep-Pak Florisil cartridge conditioned with chloroform-methanol-triethylamine. A final evaporation step under nitrogen took place before HPLC analysis. An octadecylsilane column with mobile phases of acetonitrile-water with an ion-pair reagent and UV detection was used. Positive results were verified by gas chromatograph-mass spectrometry in the electron-impact or positive or negative chemical-ionization mode. The authors claimed that the limit of detection ranged from 20 to 50 ng/g with a recovery of 66 to 87% (standard deviations from 2.2 to 11.6) except for oxfendazole which had recoveries between 40-45% in kidney and liver. The sensitivity could not be verified since control tissue chromatograms were not provided. Disadvantages of this procedure were the time consuming extractions and drying steps, use of highly toxic halogenated solvents, the additional expense of two SPE cartridges, and the inability to resolve all eight benzimidazoles in a single LC system. The major advantage was high precision.

A liquid chromatographic method using UV detection for measuring eight benzimidazoles in bovine, ovine, and swine muscle and liver was developed (Wilson *et al.* 1991). After extraction with ethyl acetate, evaporation, and final extraction with hexane, ethanol, and hydrochloric acid, samples were separated by reverse-phase liquid chromatography, using methanol and aqueous buffer as the mobile phase. Presumptive positive samples were confirmed by selected ion monitoring electron-impact gas chromatography/mass spectrometry. At 100 ng/g, overall recovery averaged 92% in liver tissue and 88% in muscle tissue for calves, swine, and sheep. Standard deviations for mean % recovery for all benzimidazoles at 50, 100, and 200 ng/g ranged from 15.3 to 23.0. The limit of detection was 50 ng/g. The major disadvantage of this method was lack of precision.

APPRAISAL

Information was provided on the metabolism of thiabendazole and the depletion of residues of thiabendazole from the edible tissues of cattle, sheep, goats and swine.

Residue depletion studies have shown thiabendazole is rapidly metabolized and excreted in all animal species and concentrations of the drug and its metabolites in tissue and excreta decrease rapidly to control levels. The major metabolite is 5-hydroxythiabendazole, generally found as its glucuronide or sulfate ester.

<u>Cattle</u> - No detectable residues of thiabendazole were found in liver, kidney, and muscle of cattle 3 days following oral doses of 50 or 110 mg/kg body weight thiabendazole. Residue levels in fat tissue approximate those found in muscle tissue.

In lactating animals, approximately 0.1 per cent of an oral dose was detectable in milk within 60 hours. Thiabendazole and its 5-hydroxythiabendazole were not detectable in the milk 60 hours after oral doses of 66, 110 or 220 mg/kg body weight.

<u>Sheep</u> - Seven days after oral administration of 82 and 100 mg/kg body weight doses of thiabendazole for sheep, no residues of the drug were found in muscle, liver and kidney.

<u>Goats</u> - Radioactive residue levels in goats which received labeled thiabendazole showed no drug residues 30 days after oral administration of 50 or 150 mg/kg body weight. Twenty-four hours after dosing with 50 mg/kg body weight only liver and kidney had detectable residues of 1.1 and 2.7 mg/kg, respectively. At 17 days post dose, no residue was found in the kidney while a residue of 0.2 mg/kg remained in the liver.

<u>Swine</u> - No residues of thiabendazole or related metabolites were found in swine tissues 7 days following a single oral dose of 100 mg thiabendazole per kg body weight.

When thiabendazole was administered to swine in the feed at 40 mg/kg body weight for two weeks, no residues of the drug or its metabolites were found in muscle, liver, kidney or fat after 7 days withdrawal, and only minute amounts (0, 0.12, 0.19, 0.17 mg/kg respectively) at a two day withdrawal period.

The following information was utilized in setting MRLs for thiabendazole:

An ADI of 0-100 μg/kg of body weight was established. This would result in a maximum ADI of 6 mg for a 60 kg human.

The total residues of thiabendazole can be approximated by the sum of thiabendazole and 5-hydroxythiabendazole and its conjugates.

The sum of the residue levels of thiabendazole and 5-hydroxythiabendazole depletes to below 0.1 mg/kg in all tissues and milk of animals within a few days of withdrawal. Assuming a total daily food intake from edible tissues and milk containing 0.1 mg/kg of thiabendazole residues, the theoretical maximum daily intake would be 0.2 mg.

{(0.1 mg/kg x 0.5 kg tissue) + (0.1 mg/kg x 1.5 kg of milk) = 0.2 mg

The theoretical maximum daily intake of 0.2 mg of thiabendazole of veterinary origin is much less than the value of 1.412 mg obtained from other agricultural uses of thiabendazole. The calculation of the latter figure was based on the Codex Maximum Residue Limits of thiabendazole in major foods and the estimated average daily global intake of these commodities. The theoretical maximum daily intake from both uses of thiabendazole utilizes 27% of the ADI.

The JMPR has set MRLs for the edible tissues of cattle, goats, horses, pigs and sheep at 0.1 mg/kg on the sum of the thiabendazole and 5-hydroxythiabendazole.

The Committee recommends MRLs for thiabendazole of 100 µg/kg for all edible tissues of cattle, goats, pigs and sheep and milk of cattle and goats. The marker residue is the sum of thiabendazole and 5-hydroxythiabendazole.

REFERENCES

Anonymous. 1981. Thiabendazole: Summary of Safety Studies. Submitted to FAO by Merck, Sharp, and Dohme.

Batty, A.F., Jones, E.M., Drewery, G., Cannon, M., and Goodwin, R. 1985. Final report, ASR 11532, November 19, 1985. Submitted to FAO by Merck, Sharp, and Dohme.

Marti, A.M., Mooser, A.E., and Koch, H. 1990. Determination of benzimidazole anthelmintics in meat samples. J. Chromat., **498,** 145-157.

Predmore, L. and Justin, J. 1987. Feeding study in lactating cattle with thiabendazole. Laboratory project #35253, April 15, 1987. Submitted to FAO by Merck, Sharp, and Dohme.

Prichard, R.K., Hennessy, D.R., Steel, J.W., and Lacey, E. 1985. Metabolite concentrations in plasma following treatment of cattle with five anthelmintics. Research Vet. Sci., **39,** 173-178.

Prichard, R.K., Steel, J.W. and Hennessy, D.R. 1981. Fenbendazole and thiabendazole in cattle: partition of gastrointestinal absorption and pharmacokinetic behavior. J. Vet. Pharmacol. Therap., **4,** 295-304.

Robinson, H.J., Brightenback, G.E., Cuckler, A.C. and Tocco, D.J. 1963. Thiabendazole: Milk residue studies in dairy cattle. November 11, 1963. Submitted to FAO by Merck, Sharp, and Dohme.

Tocco, D.J. 1960. Thiabendazole: Tissue residues in sheep. Progres report. March-April 1960. Submitted to FAO by Merck, Sharp, and Dohme.

Tocco, D.J., Buhs, R.P., Brown, H.D., Matzuk, A.R., Mertel, H.E., Harman, R.E. and Trenner, N.R. 1964. The metabolic fate of thiabendazole in sheep. J. Med. Chem., **7,** 399-405.

Tocco, D.J., Egerton, J.R., Bowers, W., Christensen, V.W. and Rosenblum, C.J. 1965. Absorption, metabolism and elimination of thiabendazole in farm animals and a method for its estimation in biological materials. J. Pharmacol. Exp. Therap., **149,** 264-271.

Tocco, D.J., Rosenblum, C., Martin, C.M. and Robinson, H.G. 1966. Absorption, metabolism and excretion of thiabendazole in man and laboratory animals. Toxicol. Appl. Pharmacol., **9,** 31-39.

Weir, A.J. 1987. Measurements of benzimidizoles and their metabolites in animal tissues. Chapter 9. Studies with thiabendazole. Ph.D. Thesis, Dept. Vet. Pharmacology, Univ. Glasgow. Submitted to FAO by Merck, Sharp, and Dohme.

Weir, A.J. and Bogan, J.A. 1985. Benzimidazole residues in liver and muscle of cattle and sheep. Proc. 3rd. Congress EAVPT, Ghent, Belgium.

Wilson, R.T. Groneck, J.M., Henry, A.C., and Rowe, L.D. 1991. Multiresidue assay for benzimidazole anthelmintics by liquid chromatography and confirmation by gas chromatography/selected-ion monitoring electron impact mass spectrometry. J. Assoc. Off. Anal. Chem., **74,** 56-67.

TRICLABENDAZOLE

IDENTITY

Chemical name: Triclabendazole

CAS Number: 68786-66-3

CAS Nomenclature: 5-Chloro-6-(2,3-dichlorophenoxy)-2-methylthio-1H-benzimidazole
6-Chloro-5-(2,3-dichlorophenoxy)-2-methylthio-benzimidazole

Synonyms: FASINEX®, FASCINEX®, FANEX®, SOFOREN®, with levamisole: ENDEX®, COMBINEX®, PARSIFAL®

Structural formula:

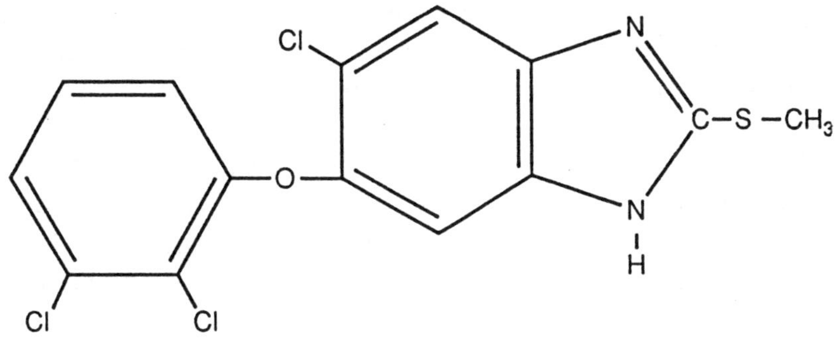

Molecular formula: $C_{14}H_{9}Cl_{3}N_{2}OS$

Molecular weight: 359.66

OTHER INFORMATION ON IDENTITY AND PROPERTIES

Pure Active Ingredient

Appearance: White, fine crystalline powder, odorless to at most a very slight odor.

Melting point: 175°C (α-modification), 162°C (β-modification)

Solubility: Readily soluble in tetrahydrofuran, cyclohexanone (45.0%), acetone (16.0%), isopropanol (12.5%), n-octanol (17.5%)

Soluble in methanol (5.5%)
Less soluble in dichloromethane
Sparingly soluble in chloroform, toluene (0.9%), xylene (0.8%), ethyl acetate
Virtually insoluble in water, hexane

Octanol/water partition coefficient: 1.75 x 10^6 cal

RESIDUES IN FOOD AND THEIR EVALUATION

CONDITIONS OF USE

General

Triclabendazole is a member of a well-known and widely used chemical class of compounds known as the benzimidazoles. It is related in chemical structure and pharmacological properties to other compounds such as thiabendazole, fenbendazole, oxibendazole, mebendazole and febantel.

Triclabendazole is an anthelmintic for the treatment and control of early immature and immature parenchymal stages and the adult bile duct stage of liver fluke infections in cattle, buffalo, sheep and goats. Triclabendazole has a narrow spectrum of activity concentrated against *Fasciola hepatica* and *F. gigantea*. Efficacy has also been described and confirmed against *Fascioloides magna* and *Paragonimus*. Triclabendazole is not active against nematodes. The recommended therapeutic dose for cattle and buffalo is 12 mg triclabendazole/kg body weight. The recommended therapeutic dose of sheep and goats is 10 mg triclabendazole/kg body weight. Treatments are repeated at 8 - 10 week intervals throughout the fluke season. Treatment in the spring serves to lessen the pasture infestation in the following autumn. For acute/subacute outbreaks, animals should be treated immediately following diagnosis. Flocks of sheep and goats should then receive repeated treatments at intervals of 5 weeks. Cattle and buffalo should receive a second treatment 6 weeks after initial diagnosis and treatment. All newly arrived animals should be treated before joining the flock/herd.

Dosages

Several formulations of triclabendazole have been developed for the treatment of food producing animals. These formulations include suspensions (5% for sheep and goats; 10% and 12%[Australia] for cattle and buffalo) and tablets (250 mg triclabendazole for sheep and goats; 900 mg triclabendazole for cattle and buffalo). Additionally, triclabendazole is available as a suspension in combination with levamisole (5% triclabendazole with 3.75% levamisole for sheep [8.75%]; 12% triclabendazole with 7.5% levamisole for cattle [19.5%]).

METABOLISM

General

The absorption, distribution, metabolism and excretion of triclabendazole have been extensively studied and are qualitatively similar in both cattle and sheep. Following oral administration, a portion of triclabendazole is absorbed from the gastrointestinal tract. Following absorption, circulating levels of triclabendazole and its metabolites are higher than those produced by the same dose of fenbendazole or albendazole. This is attributed principally to strong protein binding and, to a lesser extent, to reduced absorption of fenbendazole and albendazole (Mohammed-Ali et al. 1986). The nonabsorbed triclabendazole is excreted in the feces as unchanged drug or as unidentified metabolites.

Absorbed triclabendazole which enters the circulation is rapidly metabolized by the liver (Strong et al. 1982a). Parent material is generally not detected in the blood following oral administration (Bull et Shume 1984). Metabolism proceeds via two routes: rapid oxidation of the methyl thiol group to the sulfoxide followed by a relatively slow oxidation of the sulfoxide to the sulfone and 4-hydroxylation of the dichlorophenoxy ring with direct secretion into the bile. Disappearance of parent triclabendazole is much more rapid than the appearance of the sulfoxide metabolite. This suggests temporary binding of the triclabendazole to tissues during conversion to the sulfoxide with subsequent release of the sulfoxide metabolite into the systemic circulation (Hennessy et al. 1987). Circulating sulfoxide and sulfone metabolites are bound to plasma albumin with some excretion in bile. Five identified metabolites account for approximately 40-60% of the administered dose. The same metabolites are identified in the feces of rats, sheep and goats. There are, however, quantitative differences in the relative proportions of metabolites between the three species (Hamböck 1983).

Elimination of the compound is virtually complete by 10 days after administration (Bull et Shume 1981). Excretion of the absorbed material is principally via the bile. Urinary excretion accounts for only a small portion of the dose.

Rat

Following oral administration of ^{14}C-triclabendazole (0.52 mg/kg and 25.3 mg/kg) in the rat, 6% of the radioactivity is recovered in the urine and 90% is excreted in the feces. By 49 hours after treatment of a rat with ^{14}C-triclabendazole at a dose of 4.6 mg/kg, 34% of the dose was excreted into the bile (Hamböck 1983). Altogether, more than 96% of the administered dose could be recovered from the excreta and expired air of the rats.

In balance studies in the rat, the vast majority of the orally administered dose has been excreted by 6-10 days postdosing (Mücke 1981, Reports 1991). Approximately 1% of administered dose remained in the bodies of the rats at the time of slaughter 6 days after treatment. The radioactivity was fairly evenly distributed except in fat, where none was detected. Neither dose nor sex influenced the distribution pattern.

Rabbit

Absorption and disposition of ^{14}C-triclabendazole was investigated in female rabbits following intravenous administration of 3 mg/kg and oral administration of 3 and 26 mg/kg (Reports DM 12/91 and CRBR 22/1991).

Triclabendazole was absorbed to a large extent from the gastrointestinal tract, irrespective of dose. Metabolism was rapid with little parent drug detectable in the blood. Formation of the sulfone was slower than formation of the sulfoxide.

Radioactive substances in the blood showed a biphasic decline following both intravenous and oral administration. Most of the radioactivity was cleared from the circulation within 72 hours via the bile. Excretion of radioactivity within 7 days accounted for 80-93% of the administered dose. Most of the dose was excreted in feces. Renally excreted metabolites were mainly conjugates.

Systemic exposure to the metabolites increased overproportionally to the oral dose between the 3 and 26 mg/kg doses. This phenomenon combined with high bioavailability could explain the high acute toxicity of triclabendazole in rabbits.

Dog

Concentrations of unchanged triclabendazole, sulfoxide and sulfone metabolites were measured in the plasma and urine of dogs following intravenous and oral administration of ^{14}C-triclabendazole (Report CRBR 25/91). Parent drug was rapidly cleared from the blood and converted to its sulfoxide and sulfone metabolites. The sulfoxide accounted for approximately 16% of the circulating radioactivity following both intravenous and oral administration. After oral administration of 0.5 mg/kg, systemic exposure to the sulfoxide represented 46% of that after intravenous dosing. The sulfone was slowly formed and eliminated. The proportion of sulfone in dogs was higher than in rabbits. Relative bioavailability at 5 and 40 mg/kg was similar to that after the 0.5 mg/kg dose. Renal elimination of triclabendazole and its metabolites was negligible.

Sheep and Goats

A sheep and a lactating goat were treated with labeled triclabendazole at a dose of 10 mg/kg in gelatin capsules. Approximately 2% and 3.5% of the administered dose was recovered in the urine of the treated goat and sheep, respectively. Feces of treated animals contained 97 - 101% of the administered dose (goat and sheep, respectively). Milk contained 0.5% of the administered dose. By 10 days postdosing, recovery was virtually complete (Hamböck and Strittmatter 1981 and 1982).

Pharmacokinetic parameters for total radioactivity in the blood of sheep and goat treated with ^{14}C-triclabendazole at 10 mg/kg were compared with kinetic parameters for sulfoxide and sulfone following treatment of sheep with 10 mg/kg of nonlabeled material (Hamböck 1982, Strong et al. 1983, and Bull 1985) or goats at 12 mg/kg (Kinabo and Bogan 1988). Differences between the values for the summation curve of arithmetic mean concentrations for each metabolite at each time point and total radioactivity are within the range of values found in a population of sheep.

In sheep and goats, three phases of absorption and distribution can be identified. The initial phase lasted from 0 to 48 hours after dosing. In phase 2, from 48 to 168 hours, elimination followed first order kinetics with an apparent biological half-life of 22 hours in the goat and 26 hours in the sheep. The third phase, from 168 hours on, elimination still followed first order kinetics but with an apparent biological half life of 45 hours in the sheep and 60 hours in the goat. The total ^{14}C-triclabendazole level in milk was consistently about one tenth the residue in plasma.

Balance studies in sheep and goats show that by 6 - 10 days after dosing the majority of orally administered doses have been excreted, predominantly via the feces (Hamböck and Strittmatter 1981 and 1982, Mücke 1981, Reports 1991). The five identified metabolites account for approximately 43% and 45% of the administered dose in sheep and goats, respectively. The biliary metabolites in sheep are predominantly sulfate or glucuronide conjugates of 4-OH-triclabendazole, 4-OH-triclabendazole-sulfoxide and 4-OH-triclabendazole-sulfone (Hennessy et al. 1987).

Cattle

Triclabendazole is rapidly metabolized following intravenous administration in cattle. The sulfoxide metabolite forms rapidly and reaches a maximum blood concentration 4 hours after treatment. The terminal half-life for the sulfoxide is approximately 13 hours. The sulfone is formed more slowly. Peak plasma concentrations are measured 32 hours after dosing. The terminal elimination half-life for the sulfone is calculated to be 40 hours (Bull et al. 1986).

Pig

Following oral administration of 10 mg/kg and 30 mg/kg, plasma concentrations of triclabendazole and its sulfoxide and sulfone metabolites were determined in pigs. Only at the higher dose were plasma concentrations of the parent drug detectable. The sulfoxide metabolite formed rapidly and reached maximum plasma concentrations 8 hours after drug administration. The sulfone metabolite was produced more slowly with maximum plasma concentrations occurring 12-24 hours after dosing. The sulfone also displayed a longer elimination half-life. Overall metabolism in the pig was approximately 3 times faster than in ruminants (Galtier and Alvinerie, undated).

Horse, Pony, Donkey

Horses, ponies (*Equus caballus*)and donkeys (*E. assinus*) were treated orally with 12 mg triclabendazole/kg body weight. Triclabendazole was not detected in any plasma sample (Formica 1987, Kinabo and Bogan 1987, Tournayre 1986). Sulfoxide plasma concentrations and area under the plasma concentration curve

(AUC) in the two species were similar. The sulfoxide concentration is approximately 33% of the levels achieved in goats, sheep and cattle at the same dose. The concentration and AUC for the sulfone were much lower in the donkey than in the other species (Kinabo and Bogan 1987).

TISSUE RESIDUE DEPLETION STUDIES

Radiolabeled Residue Depletion Studies

Rat

Six days following oral administration of ^{14}C-triclabendazole, rats were slaughtered and the residual radioactivity assayed. Residues in rats treated with 0.5 mg/kg were uniformly low. Residues in rats treated with 25 mg/kg were accordingly higher. There was no organ-specific retention of radiolabel and approximately 1% of the administered dose remained in the animals six days after dosing (Mücke 1981).

Sheep and Goats

A sheep and a goat were treated once orally with ^{14}C-triclabendazole at 10.12 mg/kg and 10.49 mg/kg, respectively (Giannone and Formica 1981b, Giannone and Formica 1983a). Animals were slaughtered 10 days after dosing. Residues were extracted after thorough alkaline solubilization of the tissues and partitioning into methylene chloride. Total radioactivity data are given in Table 1.

A lactating goat was treated orally with a single dose of 10.1 mg ^{14}C-triclabendazole/kg body weight. Radioactivity was determined in the blood and milk over a 240 hour period. Radioactivity in selected tissues was determined at slaughter 10 days following drug administration. Residues in the plasma and milk are shown in Table 2 (Hamböck and Strittmatter 1981). Tissue residues were comparable to those seen in Table 1.

Table 1. ^{14}C-Triclabendazole residues in the tissues of sheep and goats dosed orally at 10.49 mg/kg and 10.12 mg/kg, respectively

Animal	Sample	Total Radioactivity	Extracted Radioactivity		Nonextracted Radioactivity	
		mg/kg	mg/kg	%total	mg/kg	%total
Sheep	Muscle	0.58	0.011	1.9	0.53	91
			0.020	3.6	0.56	96
					0.56	96
	Liver	1.84	0.13	7.2	1.66	90
					1.72	93
	Kidney	1.11	0.14	12.9		
	Fat	0.09	0.012	13.0		
Goat	Muscle	0.44	0.009	2.0		
	Liver	1.00	0.075	7.5		
			0.069	6.9		
	Kidney	0.69	0.05	7.2		
	Fat	0.08	0.005	6.0		

Table 2. Concentration of radioactivity (in ppm triclabendazole equivalents) in the plasma and milk of a lactating goat treated with 10.1 mg ^{14}C-triclabendazole/kg body weight

Collection (h)	Triclabendazole eq (ppm)	
	Plasma	Milk
8	15.75	0.529
24	22.78	1.788
48	15.30	1.375
72	7.28	0.771
96	3.17	0.372
120	1.28	0.158
144	0.52	0.072
168	0.26	0.039
176	NA	0.027
192	0.15	0.020
200	NA	0.020
216	0.11	0.016
224	NA	0.014
239	0.09	0.012

A sheep was treated with 10.5 mg ^{14}C-triclabendazole/kg as a single oral dose. Radioactivity was determined in the blood for 240 hours. First order elimination resulted in half-lifes of 26 hours for the period from 48-200 hours postdosing and 45 hours for the period from 200 hours to the end of the sampling period at 240 hours postdosing. The sheep was sacrificed 10 days after dosing and the residues in selected tissues were determined. The concentration of radioactivity in the plasma is shown in Table 3 (Hamböck and Strittmatter 1982). Tissue residues were comparable to those seen in Table 1 above.

Table 3. Concentration of radioactivity (in ppm triclabendazole equivalents) in the plasma of a sheep treated with 10.5 mg ^{14}C-triclabendazole/kg body weight

Collection (h)	Triclabendazole eq (ppm)
1	0.05
4	5.16
8	13.62
24	27.04
48	22.08
72	12.14
96	6.08
120	3.00
144	1.62
168	0.71
192	0.37
216	0.22
239	0.11

Cattle

Two ruminating heifers were treated with a single oral dose of ^{14}C-triclabendazole at the rate of 12 mg/kg body weight. The animals were slaughtered at 28 and 42 days after dosing (Downs et al. 1991). Total residues are shown in Table 4.

Table 4. Concentration of radioactivity (in ppm triclabendazole equivalents) in the tissues of cattle treated with a single oral dose of ^{14}C-triclabendazole at 12 mg/kg body weight

Withdrawal (days)	Liver	Kidney	Muscle	Fat
28	0.241 ± 0.013	0.106 ± 0.016	0.131 ± 0.017	0.013 ± 0.003
42	0.093 ± 0.009	0.069 ± 0.011	0.097 ± 0.007	<0.008 ± 0.001

OTHER RESIDUE DEPLETION STUDIES

Sheep and Goats

In a lactating goat, triclabendazole and its sulfoxide and sulfone metabolites are present in the milk following oral administration of 10.12 mg triclabendazole/kg body weight. Unchanged triclabendazole is detectable in milk samples for 96 hours following dosing. Both the sulfoxide and sulfone metabolites reach their maximum concentrations in milk 24 hours after treatment and decrease thereafter (Giannone and Formica 1981a).

Sixteen sheep were treated with triclabendazole as a single oral administration at either 10 mg/kg or 15 mg/kg. "Total" residues were determined by a method that measures residues of triclabendazole and its metabolites that are oxidizable to 5-chloro-6-(2',3'-dichlorophenoxy)-benzimidazole-2-one (MR). The "total" residues are converted to triclabendazole equivalents using a conversion factor of 1.0913. Residues were determined at 2, 7, 14, 21 or 28 days for the sheep receiving the 10 mg/kg dose and at 7 and 14 days for sheep treated with 15 mg/kg (Giannone and Formica 1983a). Results of the study are shown in Table 5.

Table 5. Total residues of triclabendazole in the tissues of sheep after a single oral treatment of 10 or 15 mg/kg body weight

Treatment mg/kg	Days After Treatment	Residues (mg Triclabendazole eq/kg)			
		Muscle	Liver	Kidney	Fat
Control		<0.029	<0.047	<0.029	<0.029
10	2	1.1	3.0	2.8	1.6
		1.5	4.0	3.4	1.1
10	7	0.16	0.54	0.34	0.043
		0.19	0.66	0.42	0.050
10	14	0.17	0.46	0.35	<0.029
		0.13	0.20	0.15	<0.029
10	21	0.092	0.18	0.15	<0.029
		0.085	0.17	0.15	<0.029
10	28	0.083	0.074	0.11	<0.029
		0.14	0.18	0.12	<0.029
15	7	0.43	1.2	0.79	0.11
		0.31	1.3	0.82	0.14
15	14	0.15	0.33	0.19	0.029
		0.13	0.44	0.22	<0.029

In a second study, 18 sheep were treated with 10 mg triclabendazole/kg body weight as a single oral dose. The animals were slaughtered 2, 7, 14, 21, 28, 42 or 56 days following administration. Total residues were determined as 5-chloro-6-(2',3'-dichloropenoxy)-benzimidazole-2-one and converted to triclabendazole equivalents using a conversion factor of 1.0913 (Giannone and Formica 1983e). The residues in the tissue of sheep are shown in Table 6.

Table 6. Total residues of triclabendazole in the tissues of sheep after a single oral treatment of 10 mg/kg body weight

Days After Treatment	Residues (mg Triclabendazole eq/kg)			
	Muscle	Liver	Kidney	Fat
7	0.30	0.62	0.28	0.071
	0.19	0.49	0.40	0.061
	0.20	0.52	0.20	0.088
14	0.25	NA	0.14	<0.03
	0.15	0.24	0.14	<0.03
	0.16	0.21	0.11	<0.03
21	0.16/0.14	0.16	0.097	<0.03
	0.15	0.11	0.11	<0.03
	0.12	0.12	0.07	<0.03
28	0.13	0.070	0.052	<0.03
	<0.095	0.098	0.048	<0.03
	0.082	0.061	0.048	<0.03
42	0.036	<0.03	0.044	<0.03
	0.043	0.033	<0.03	<0.03
	0.061/0.058	<0.03	<0.03	<0.03
56	0.092	NA	<0.03	<0.03
	0.070	<0.03	<0.03	<0.03
	0.070/0.066	<0.03	<0.03	<0.03

In a study involving a single sheep dosed orally with triclabendazole at a rate of 10 mg/kg, triclabendazole and its sulfoxide and sulfone metabolites were quantified individually in the plasma. Parent drug was not detected at any time during the study. The sulfoxide metabolite peaked at 24 hours postadministration and the sulfone peaked at 48 hours after dosing. An elimination half-life of approximately 30 hours was calculated from the combined terminal elimination phase of sulfoxide plus sulfone (Alvinerie and Galtier 1986).

Twelve sheep were treated a single oral dose of a 8.75% ENDEX® suspension (10 mg triclabendazole and 7.5 mg levamisole hydrochloride) at a rate of 17.5 mg/kg body weight. Two additional heifers served as controls. Animals were slaughtered at 1, 21 and 28 days after dosing. Results are are shown in Table 7. Total residues were determined as 5-chloro-6-(2',3'-dichlorophenoxy)-benzimidazole-2-one and converted to triclabendazole equivalents using a conversion factor of 1.0913 (Lanter 1989a).

Table 7. Total residues of triclabendazole (as triclabendazole equivalents/kg) in the tissues of sheep treated with 8.75% ENDEX

Days After Treatment	Residues (mg Triclabendazole eq/kg)			
	Muscle	Liver	Kidney	Fat
Control	<0.04	<0.05	<0.04	<0.05
1	2.2	5.4	6.2	13.4
	2.1	8.9	6.2	10.7
	2.3	7.6	8.7	8.8
	1.7	7.8	6.0	7.6
21	0.16	0.25	0.17	<0.05
	0.15	0.15	0.13	<0.05
	0.15	0.24	0.12	<0.05
	0.09	0.16	0.07	<0.05
28	0.10	0.11	0.07	<0.05
	0.19	0.10	0.06	<0.05
	0.14	0.11	0.07	<0.05
	0.17	0.18	0.06	<0.05

<u>Cattle</u>

Twelve cattle were treated with a single oral dose of triclabendazole at a rate of 12 mg/kg body weight. The animals were slaughtered 2, 7, 14, 21 or 28 days following administration. Total residues were determined as 5-chloro-6-(2',3'-dichlorophenoxy)-benzimidazole-2-one and converted to triclabendazole equivalents using a conversion factor of 1.0913 (Giannone and Formica 1983c). The residues in the tissue of cattle are shown in Table 8.

Table 8. **Total residues of triclabendazole in the tissues of cattle after a single oral treatment of 12 mg/kg body weight**

Days After Treatment	Residues (mg Triclabendazole eq/kg)			
	Muscle	Liver	Kidney	Fat
Control	<0.03	<0.03	<0.046	<0.03
2	1.01	2.9	2.8	1.7
	0.74	3.6	3.3	1.9
7	0.14	0.43	0.41	0.088
	0.16	0.44	0.52	0.079
14	0.080	0.096	0.14	<0.03
	0.064	0.17	0.16	<0.03
21	0.056	0.089	0.068	<0.03
	0.065	0.12	0.092	<0.03
28	0.044	0.055	0.049	<0.03
	<0.03	0.048	0.046	<0.03

In a later study (Formica 1984), ten cattle were treated once orally with 12 mg triclabendazole/kg body weight. The animals were slaughtered 2, 7, 14, 28 or 42 days following administration. Total residues were determined as 5-chloro-6-(2',3'-dichlorophenoxy)-benzimidazole-2-oneandconvertedtotriclabendazoleequivalents using a conversion factor of 1.0913. Results are shown in Table 9.

Table 9. **Total residues of triclabendazole in the tissues of cattle after a single oral treatment of 12 mg/kg body weight**

Days After Treatment	Residues (mg Triclabendazole eq/kg)			
	Muscle	Liver	Kidney	Fat
Control	<0.04	<0.04	<0.03	<0.06
2	1.42	7.46	4.33	2.55
	1.42	4.28	4.26	2.39
7	0.34	1.0	0.70	0.11
	0.24	0.58	0.68	0.15
14	0.20	0.61	0.29	0.07
	0.19	0.35	0.28	<0.05
28	0.09	0.17	0.09	<0.06
	0.10	0.15	0.11	<0.05
42	0.11	0.07	0.08	<0.06
	0.09	0.09	0.07	<0.05

Twelve Friesian heifers were treated with a single oral dose of a 19.5% ENDEX® suspension (12 mg triclabendazole and 7.5 mg levamisole hydrochloride). Two additional heifers served as controls. Animals were slaughtered at 1, 21 and 28 days after dosing. Results are are shown in Table 10. Total residues were determined as 5-chloro-6(2',3'-dichlorophenoxy)-benzimidazole-2-one and converted to triclabendazole equivalents using a conversion factor of 1.0913 (Lanter 1989b).

Table 10. Total residues of triclabendazole (as triclabendazole equivalents/kg) in the tissues of cattle treated with 19.5% ENDEX

Days After Treatment	Residues (mg Triclabendazole eq/kg)			
	Muscle	Liver	Kidney	Fat
Control	<0.04	<0.04	<0.04	<0.04
1	1.3	6.4	5.8	3.7
	1.9	9.5	6.9	7.6
	1.3	6.3	5.4	4.6
	1.1	6.0	5.0	4.1
21	0.19	0.32	0.18	<0.04
	0.11	0.19	0.14	<0.04
	0.15	0.26	0.17	<0.04
	0.16	0.29	0.22	<0.04
28	0.11	0.15	0.11	<0.04
	0.14	0.14	0.10	<0.04
	0.13	0.12	0.08	<0.04
	0.19	0.16	0.12	<0.04

BIOAVAILABILITY

Sheep and Goats

To estimate the bioavailability of triclabendazole in sheep after oral administration, the AUC of the sulfoxide metabolite was compared after intravenous and oral dosing. The sulfoxide was used due to the rapid metabolism of parent drug to this primary metabolite. The assumption is made that intravenously administered drug is 100% available. The relative bioavailability of triclabendazole was calculated to be 90% (Strong et al. 1982a, Strong et al. 1983). Biliary and renal excretion data raise doubts about the bioavailability of the intravenously administered dose. In sheep, approximately 50% of the dose was excreted in the bile in 6 days and urinary excretion in 10 days accounted for only 2.1% of the administered dose.

This means that the real bioavailability is much lower than that calculated by comparing intravenous and oral dosing. This could be due to removal of a proportion of the intravenous dose by a specific tissue or tissues. While the appearance of triclabendazole metabolites in the plasma is a function of both absorption from the gastrointestinal tract and release of bound material, circulating levels do not directly correlate with the efficacy of triclabendazole in controlling flukes (Strong *et al.* 1982b).

Based on limited experimentation, there are no consistent differences in the absorption properties of suspension formulations containing triclabendazole at concentrations of 25 mg/ml, 50 mg/ml or 100 mg/ml (Strong et al. 1982a), in different 50 mg/ml suspension formulations (Strong et al 1982b) or in bolus vs. drench preparations (Bowen et al. 1984). Differences in plasma levels of triclabendazole metabolites which were observed appear to be the result of interanimal variability and not esophageal groove reflex in treated sheep (Strong et al. 1983). In general, changes in crystal form or particle size distribution do not affect the plasma kinetic profiles of the triclabendazole metabolites (Strong et al. 1986).

METHODS OF ANALYSIS FOR RESIDUES IN TISSUES

Triclabendazole residues can be measured by a high performance liquid chromatograph (HPLC) method using ultraviolet absorbance detection. The method measures residues of triclabendazole with are hydrolyzable and oxidizable to 5-chloro-6-(2',3'-dichlorophenoxy)-benzimidazole-2-one (MR). Tissue samples are hydrolyzed under alkaline conditions at 90-100°C and the entire hydrolysate is extracted with methylene chloride under acidic conditions. Following evaporation of the methylene chloride, lipid material is removed by dissolving the residue in hexane and partitioning with acetonitrile. The acetonitrile is evaporated and the residue is dissolved in a mixture of acetic acid/ethanol and oxidized overnight with hydrogen peroxide at 90°C. The mixture is acidified and MR is partitioned into methylene chloride. Further clean up is carried out on a Silica Gel column followed by a C_{18} SEP-PAK column prior to HPLC on a 10 μm LiChrosphere Si 100 column, 25 cm x 4.6 mm i.d. A mobile phase consisting of a mixture of dichloromethane/hexane/anhydrous ethanol/glacial acetic acid (700/300/50/4) at a flow rate of 1.5 cm^3/min is used to effect separation. Effluent is monitored at 295 nm (Giannone and Formica 1983b). Alternatively, the SEP-PAK clean up can be omitted by the use of column switching with two LiChrosphere Si 100 columns (Giannone and Formica 1983f). The limit of detection is 4 ng corresponding to 0.027 mg MR/kg or 0.03 mg triclabendazole/kg (conversion factor 1.0913). Recoveries from spiked samples in tissues of cattle and sheep are shown in Table 11.

Table 11. Recoveries (%) of MR in tissues of sheep and cattle

Tissue	Fortification level mg/kg	Recoveries after SEP-PAK		Recoveries after Column Switching
		Cattle	Sheep	Sheep
Muscle	0.1	109	85/69/95	97/95
	0.5	76	87/67/70/74	72/79
Kidney	0.1	80	80/73/83/74	89/98
	0.5	70	77/72/75/67/75	75/76
Liver	0.1	41	82/76/68/68	67/75
	0.5	77	58/70/60/66	76/79
Fat	0.1	69	53	71/73/68
	0.5	55	69	54/60/61

Modification of the method to use HPLC column 2 packed with 10μm Lichrosorb Diol instead of LiChrosphere Si 100 permits the determination of MR in the tissues of sheep treated with 8.75% ENDEX (Lanter 1989a) or cattle treated with 19.5% ENDEX (Lanter 1989b). The practical limit of detection is 0.04-0.05 mg/kg as CGA 89317 (triclabendazole).

Using a mobile phase of hexane/ethanol/glacial acetic acid (500:50:0.6, v/v/v) on a 5μm Partisil silica gel column, triclabendazole and its sulfoxide and sulfone metabolites are quantified from a plasma matrix following ethyl acetate extraction. The HPLC system employs an ultraviolet detector set at 215 nm and a solvent flow rate of 1.5 ml/min. Oxfendazole is used as an internal standard. The system is linear from 0.1-4.0 μg/ml and has a detection limit of 50 ng/ml for all products (Alvinerie and Galtier 1986).

A reversed-phase HPLC method using a 10μm microBondapak column and a solvent system containing methanol/water/reagent 1(120 ml glacial acetic acid + 200 g ammonium acetate q.s. 1 l)/chloroform (750:200:25:10, v/v/v/v) also provides quantification of triclabendazole and its metabolites. Detection is ultraviolet at 300 nm with a flow rate of 1 ml/min. The limit of detection is 0.1 mg/l (Bull and Shume 1987a).

A similar method is employed for the simultaneous detection of fenbendazole, its sulfoxide and sulfone metabolites and the corresponding metabolites of triclabendazole. Using a reversed-phase column, a solvent system containing acetonitrile/0.04M diammonium hydrogen orthophosphate (41:59, v/v) adjusted to pH 7.5-7.6 effects the separation. The system is linear over a range of 5-500 ng with a 10 ng/ml limit of determination in plasma (Bull and Shume 1987b).

In an earlier method for the simultaneous determination of fenbendazole, its sulfoxide and sulfone metabolites and the corresponding metabolites of triclabendazole, a 5μm Hypersil SAS (mixed C_2-, C_4-, C_6-silica) column was used. A mobile phase containing 0.005M phosphoric acid (adjusted to pH 5.9 with tetraethylammonium hydroxide solution)/ acetonitrile (70:30) at a flow rate of 2.0 ml/min was used for the separation. The effluent was monitored at 300 nm. The system is linear over the range of 20-1000 ng/ml in plasma for fenbendazole and its metabolites and 50-1000 ng/m for the triclabendazole metabolites. The limit of determination is stated to be 10 ng/ml for the fenbendazole metabolites, 15 ng/ml for parent fenbendazole, and 20 ng/ml for the triclabendazole metabolites (Lehr and Damm 1986).

A solid phase extraction procedure is also reported for sample preparation prior to HPLC analysis with fluorescence detection. Blood samples from goats, horses, ponies and donkeys and milk samples from goats were precipitated with acetone. The resultant supernatant is mixed with water and loaded onto preconditioned SEP-PAK cartridge. A 5μm ODS-Hypersil column with a mobile phase of 0.13M ammonium acetate buffer (pH 6.7)/methanol (30:70, v/v) was used to effect separation. Excitation and emission wavelengths were 300 nm and 676 nm, respectively. Detection limits were 0.02 μg/ml for triclabendazole sulfone and 0.04 μg/ml for triclabendazole sulfoxide. Recovery of triclabendazole and its sulfoxide and sulfone metabolites from plasma and milk ranged from 76-92% (Kinabo and Bogan 1987 and 1988).

An extraction method was validated to determine the relationship of residues resulting from chemical extraction to "true" total residues determined using combustion analysis and liquid scintillation. Tissue samples were macerated with methanol and shaken for 30 minutes. An aliquot of the clear extract was taken for scintillation counting. Only 2-13% of the total radioactivity was extracted from the tissue samples. The method is considered not valid for the determination of total residues in tissue samples (Giannone and Formica 1981b).

The HPLC method was validated to determine the relationship of residues determined by HPLC-UV to "true" total residues. Tissue samples were collected from a goat treated with ^{14}C-triclabendazole ten days following treatment. Total radioactivity was determined via liquid scintillation counting after combustion. The SEP-PAK clean up was not included in the tissue sample preparation and only muscle tissue was analyzed. Approximately 32-38% of the total radioactivity in goat muscle can be determined using the HPLC-UV method (Giannone and Formica 1983d).

Blood and milk were collected from a goat treated with ^{14}C-triclabendazole. Milk and blood samples were prepared by precipitation of proteins with acetone followed by partitioning into dichloromethane. Samples were evaporated to dryness. Milk samples were dissolved in hexane and cleaned up with acetonitrile. After evaporation of the acetonitrile, samples were cleaned up and separated on a degassed alumina column prior to final HPLC-UV analysis. Blood samples were prepared similarly but the hexane/acetonitrile partition step was eliminated. Residues of triclabendazole and its metabolites account for approximately 54-79% of the radioactivity in milk and 100% of the radioactivity in blood. The limit of determination in blood and milk is 0.005 mg/kg (Giannone and Formica 1981a).

APPRAISAL

The absorption, distribution, metabolism and excretion of triclabendazole have been studied and are qualitatively similar in both cattle and sheep. As with several other benzimidazoles, the use of triclabendazole in food producing animals results in a large portion of the total residue being bound to endogenous tissue. The proportion of bound residue to total residue increases with increasing withdrawal periods. The marker residue for triclabendazole is 5-chloro-6-(2′,3′-dichlorophenoxy)-benzimidazole-2-one (MR). MR results when common fragments of triclabendazole-related residues are hydrolyzed under alkaline conditions at 90-100°C. As the marker residue does not measure total residues, the ratio for the marker residue and the total residue needs to be determined for each species. The marker residue levels are converted to triclabendazole equivalents using a conversion factor of 1.09.

Cattle - In three separate residue depletion studies cattle were dosed with triclabendazole at 12 mg/kg body weight. The residues of MR were determined in the edible tissues at various withdrawal times. A common withdrawal time for all three studies was 28 days. The average values (n=8) of MR at the 28 day withdrawal time were 0.12, 0.07, 0.11 and 0.05 mg/kg in liver, kidney, muscle and fat. These values represent 50, 66, 84 and >100% of the total residue in the respective tissues at a withdrawal time of 28 days.

Sheep. - In two separate residue depletion studies sheep were dosed with triclabendazole at 10 mg/kg body weight. The residues of MR were determined in the edible tissues at various withdrawal times. Common withdrawal times for both studies were 7, 14 and 28 days. Combining the residue levels at 7 and 14 days to approximate the residue levels at 10 days in the radiolabel study, the average values (n=10 for kidney and muscle; n=9 for liver) of MR were 0.44, 0.25, 0.19 and 0.04 mg/kg in liver, kidney, muscle and fat. These values represent 24, 23, 33 and 51% of the triclabendazole-related total residues in the respective tissues. Using these percentages and residue concentrations of MR at 28 days withdrawal of 0.097, 0.076, 0.11 and <0.03 mg/kg in the respective tissue, the concentration of total triclabendazole-related residues is approximated to be 159 μg.

The following information was utilized in setting the MRLs for triclabendazole:

An ADI of 0-3 μg/kg of body weight was established. This would result in a maximum ADI of 180 μg for a 60 kg human.

Considering the vigorous extraction conditions of the method for MR, the method likely measures more residues than those usually defined as extractable residues. However, the method does not measure total residues.

Recommended MRLs for Triclabendazole in Cattle

Tissue	Concentration of MR at Day 28 Withdrawal, μg/kg 12 mg/kg oral dose	Total Residue Consumed μg(a)	Recommended MRL μg/kg MR	Theoretical Maximum Daily Intake μg(a)
Muscle	110(131)b	39	200(238)b	71
Liver	120(240)c	24	300(600)c	60
Kidney	70(106)d	5	300(454)d	23
Fat	50	2	100	5
	Total	70		159

a) Based on a daily intake of 0.3 kg muscle, 0.1 kg liver, 0.05 kg kidney and fat.
b) Adjusted observed value by 84% to estimate total residues.
c) Adjusted observed value by 50% to estimate total residues.
d) Adjusted observed value by 66% to estimate total residues.

Recommended MRLs for Triclabendazole in Sheep

Using the residue data at 28 days withdrawal for sheep and assuming the ratio of marker residue to total residue at 28 days is approximated by the ratio at 10 days withdrawal, the dietary intake for all triclabendazole related residues at 28 days withdrawal is approximately 159 μg.

Tissue	Concentration of MR at Day 28 Withdrawal, μg/kg 10 mg/kg oral dose	Total Residue Consumed μg(a)	Recommended MRL μg/kg MR	Theoretical Maximum Daily Intake μg(a)
Muscle	110(333)b	100	100(303)b	91
Liver	97(404)c	40	100(417)c	42
Kidney	76(330)d	16	100(435)d	22
Fat	<30(59)e	3	100(196)e	10
	Total	159		165

a) Based on a daily intake of 0.3 kg muscle, 0.1 kg liver, 0.05 kg kidney and fat.
b) Adjusted observed value by 33% to estimate total residues.
c) Adjusted observed value by 24% to estimate total residues.
d) Adjusted observed value by 23% to estimate total residues.
e) Adjusted observed value by 51% to estimate total residues.

Additional data are required if the MRLs for triclabendazole in sheep are to be increased. A more accurate estimate of the total residues in edible tissues of sheep is needed. Also, the ratio of total residue concentrations to the marker residue concentrations is needed. Considering that the recommended MRLs require all of the ADI at 28 days, bioavailability studies on the bound residue of triclabendazole may be needed to reduce the amount of residue of toxicological concern.

REFERENCES

Alvinerie, M., and Galtier, P. 1986. Assay of triclabendazole and its main metabolites in plasma by high-performance liquid chromatography. J. Chromatogr. (Biomed. Appl.), **374**,409-414.

Bowen, F. L., Allison, J. R., and Strong, M. B. 1984. A comparison of the efficacy of Fasinex formulated as a bolus or as a liquid drench suspension against two week old infections of Fasciola hepatica in cattle. CIBA-GEIGY Australia Ltd. R & D Technical Report 84/10/1048. Submitted to FAO by CIBA-GEIGY, Ltd., Basel, Switzerland.

Bull, M. S. 1985. Pharmacokinetics of triclabendazole capsules in sheep. CIBA-GEIGY Ltd. R & D Memorandum 85/10/1048. Submitted to FAO by CIBA-GEIGY, Ltd., Basel, Switzerland.

Bull, M. S., and Shume, G. R. 1981. The determination of residues of CGA 89317 and its metabolites CGA 110752 and CGA 110753 in the fat and tissues of sheep dosed orally with CGA 89317 at 10 mg a.i./kg. CIBA-GEIGY Australia Ltd. R & D Technical Report 81/2/847. Submitted to FAO by CIBA-GEIGY, Ltd., Basel, Switzerland.

Bull, M. S. and Shume, G. R. 1984. The levels of triclabendazole, fenbendazole and their associated sulphoxide and sulphone metabolites in sheep serum following oral treatment with Fasinex and Pancur alone and in a formulation combination. CIBA-GEIGY Australia Ltd. R & D Technical Report 84/4/992. Submitted to FAO by CIBA-GEIGY, Ltd., Basel, Switzerland.

Bull, M. S., and Shume, G. R. E. 1987a. A rapid high-performance liquid chromatographic procedure for the determination of triclabendazole and its metabolites in sheep plasma. J. Pharm. Biomed. Anal., **5**, 527-531.

Bull, M. S., and Shume, G. R. E. 1987b. Simultaneous determination of fenbendazole, its sulphoxide and sulphone metabolites with the corresponding metabolites of triclabendazole in the plasma of sheep and cattle by high-performance liquid chromatography. J. Pharm. Biomed. Anal., **5**, 501-508.

Bull, M. S., Bowen, F. L., and Kearney, E. M. 1986. The bioavailability of triclabendazole and its sulphoxide metabolite in cattle. CIBA-GEIGY Australia Ltd., R & D Technical Report 86/12/1099. Submitted to FAO by CIBA-GEIGY, Ltd., Basel, Switzerland.

Downs, J. H., Marsh, J. D., and Krautter, G. R. 1991. Depletion of total drug-related residues in tissues of beef cattle treated with [14C] triclabendazole (Pilot Study). PTRL East Inc. July 26, 1991. Submitted to FAO by CIBA-GEIGY, Ltd., Basel, Switzerland.

Formica, G. 1984. Determination of total residues of CGA 89317 in cattle muscle, liver, kidney and fat after a single oral treatment at a rate of 12 mg a.i./kg body weight. CIBA-GEIGY Ltd., Basel, Switzerland, Residue Report RVA 4023/83, August 20, 1984. Submitted to FAO by CIBA-GEIGY, Ltd., Basel, Switzerland.

Formica, G. 1987. Residue determination of parent compound and its oxidized metabolites CGA 110752 and CGA 110753 in pony plasma after one oral medication either with FASINEX 10% suspension or FASINEX tablets. CIBA-GEIGY Ltd., Basel, Switzerland, Analysis Report 906/87, July 7, 1987. Submitted to FAO by CIBA-GEIGY, Ltd., Basel, Switzerland.

Galtier, P. and Alvinerie, M. (undated) Report on trials to study the pharmacokinetics of triclabendazole in the pig. INRA Station de Pharmacologie-Toxicologie, Toulouse, France. Submitted to FAO by CIBA-GEIGY, Ltd., Basel, Switzerland.

Giannone, C. and Formica, G. 1981a. CGA 89317, validation of method REM 6/81 (residue determination of parent compound and its metabolites in milk and blood by high performance liquid chromatography). CIBA-GEIGY Ltd., Basel, Switzerland, Report SPR 12/81, June 5, 1981. Submitted to FAO by CIBA-GEIGY, Ltd., Basel, Switzerland.

Giannone, C. and Formica, G. 1981b. Validation of R & D analytical method No. 186. Australia. CIBA-GEIGY Ltd., Basel, Switzerland. Report SPR 17/81, July 15, 1981. Submitted to FAO by CIBA-GEIGY, Ltd., Basel, Switzerland.

Giannone, C. and Formica, G. 1983a. Determination of total residues of CGA 89317 in sheep muscle, liver, kidney and fat after a single oral treatment at a rate of 10 mg/kg or 15 mg/kg body weight. CIBA-GEIGY Ltd., Basel, Switzerland, Residue Report RVA 4005/82, May 5, 1983. Submitted to FAO by CIBA-GEIGY, Ltd., Basel, Switzerland.

Giannone, C. and Formica, G. 1983b. CGA 89317 - Determination of total residues in tissues and fat of sheep and cattle. CIBA-GEIGY Ltd., Basel, Switzerland, Method REM 3/83, June 1, 1983. Submitted to FAO by CIBA-GEIGY, Ltd., Basel, Switzerland.

Giannone, C. and Formica, G. 1983c. Determination of total residues of CGA 89317 in cattle muscle, liver, kidney and fat after a single oral treatment at a rate of 12 mg a.i./kg body weight. CIBA-GEIGY Ltd., Basel, Switzerland, Residue Report RVA 4006/82, June 3, 1983. Submitted to FAO by CIBA-GEIGY, Ltd., Basel, Switzerland.

Giannone, C. and Formica, G. 1983d. Validation of method REM 3/83 (Determination of total residues in tissues and fat of sheep and cattle.) CIBA-GEIGY Ltd., Basel, Switzerland, Residue Report SPR 11/83, June 3, 1983. Submitted to FAO by CIBA-GEIGY, Ltd., Basel, Switzerland.

Giannone, C. and Formica, G. 1983e. Determination of total residues of CGA 89317 in sheep muscle, liver, kidney and fat after a single oral treatment at a rate of 10 mg/kg body weight. CIBA-GEIGY Ltd., Basel, Switzerland, Residue Report RVA 4002/83, December 1, 1983. Submitted to FAO by CIBA-GEIGY, Ltd., Basel, Switzerland.

Giannone, C. and Formica, G. 1983f. Determination of total residues in animal tissues and fat. CIBA-GEIGY Ltd., Basel, Switzerland, Method REM 15/83, December 7, 1983. Submitted to FAO by CIBA-GEIGY, Ltd., Basel, Switzerland.

Hamböck, H. 1982. Characterization of tissue residues of CGA 89371 in sheep and goat. CIBA-GEIGY Ltd., Basel, Switzerland, Project Report 50/82. Submitted to FAO by CIBA-GEIGY, Ltd., Basel, Switzerland.

Hamböck, H. 1983. The metabolic fate of CGA 89317 in sheep, rat and the lactating goat. CIBA-GEIGY Ltd., Basel, Switzerland, AG 2.52 Project Report 41/83, December 12, 1983. Submitted to FAO by CIBA-GEIGY, Ltd., Basel, Switzerland.

Hamböck, H. and Strittmatter, J. 1981. Distribution, degradation and excretion of CGA 89317 in the lactating goat. CIBA-GEIGY Ltd., Basel, Switzerland, AG 2.52 Project Report 34/81, November 10, 1981. Submitted to FAO by CIBA-GEIGY, Ltd., Basel, Switzerland.

Hamböck, H. and Strittmatter, J. 1982. Distribution, degradation and excretion of CGA 89317 in sheep. CIBA-GEIGY Ltd., Basel, Switzerland, AG 2.52 Project Report 10/82, April 19, 1982. Submitted to FAO by CIBA-GEIGY, Ltd., Basel, Switzerland.

Hennessy, D. R., Lacey, E., Steel, J. W., and Pritchard, R. K. 1987. The kinetics of triclabendazole disposition in sheep. J. Vet. Pharmacol. Therap., **10**, **64-72.**

Kinabo, L. D. B. and Bogan, J. A. 1987. Pharmacokinetics of triclabendazole in horses, ponies and donkeys. October 12, 1987. Submitted to FAO by CIBA-GEIGY, Ltd., Basel, Switzerland. [also: Equine Veterinary J.(1989)21,305-307.]

Kinabo, L. D. B. and Bogan, J. A. 1988. Pharmacokinetics and efficacy of triclabendazole in goats with induced fascioliasis. J. Vet. Pharmacol. Ther., (1988)11,254-259.

Lanter, F. 1989a. Determination of total residues in muscle, liver, kidney and fat after a single oral treatment with Endex 8.75% suspension at a dose rate of 17.5 mg/kg body weight (i.e. 10 mg/kg triclabendazole and 7.5 mg/kg levamisole hydrochloride). CIBA-GEIGY Ltd., Basel, Switzerland, AG 2.53 Residue Report 4001/89, May 10, 1989. Submitted to FAO by CIBA-GEIGY, Ltd., Basel, Switzerland.

Lanter, F. 1989b. Determination of total residues in muscle, liver, kidney and fat after a single oral treatment with Endex 19.5% suspension at a dose rate of 19.5 mg/kg body weight (i.e. 12 mg/kg triclabendazole and 7.5 mg/kg levamisole hydrochloride). CIBA-GEIGY Ltd., Basel, Switzerland, AG 2.53 Residue Report 4002/89, July 6, 1989. Submitted to FAO by CIBA-GEIGY, Ltd., Basel, Switzerland.

Lehr, K. H., and Damm, P. 1986. Simultaneous determination of fenbendazole and its two metabolites and two triclabendazole metabolites in the plasma by high-performance liquid chromatography. J. Chromatogr. (Biomed. Appl.), **382**,355-360.

Mohammed-Ali, N. A. K., Bogan, J. A., Marriner, S. E., and Richards, R. J. 1986. Pharmacokinetics of triclabendazole alone or in combination with fenbendazole in sheep. J. vet. Pharmacol. Therap., **9**,442-445.

Mücke, W. 1981. Distribution, degradation and excretion of CGA 89317 in the rat. CIBA-GEIGY Ltd., Basel, Switzerland, AG 2.52 Project Report 27/81, August 24, 1981. Submitted to FAO by CIBA-GEIGY, Ltd., Basel, Switzerland.

Report C. R. B. R. 25 1991. Kinetics in dogs and rats. Laboratoires CIBA-GEIGY, Rueil Malmaison France, May 14, 1991. Submitted to FAO by CIBA-GEIGY, Ltd., Basel, Switzerland.

Report C. R. B. R. 22 1991. Kinetics in female rabbits. Laboratoires CIBA-GEIGY, Rueil Malmaison France, May 14, 1991. Submitted to FAO by CIBA-GEIGY, Ltd., Basel, Switzerland.

Report D. M. 12 1991. CGP 23030, triclabendazole, FASINEX. Absorption and disposition studies in female rabbits. CIBA-GEIGY, Ltd., Basel, Switzerland. Pharma Research and Development, May 2, 1991. Submitted to FAO by CIBA-GEIGY, Ltd., Basel, Switzerland.

Strong, M. B., Bull, M. S., and Shume, G. 1982a. Pharmacokinetic studies carried out with CGA 89317 and its metabolites CGA 110752 and CGA 110753 in sheep. CIBA-GEIGY Australia Ltd., R & D Technical Report 82/7/916. Submitted to FAO by CIBA-GEIGY, Ltd., Basel, Switzerland.

Strong, M. B., Bull, M. S., and Shume, G. 1982b. Pharmacokinetic studies carried out with CGA 89317 and its metabolites in the plasma of sheep infected with 4 week old fluke. CIBA-GEIGY Australia Ltd., R & D Technical Report 82/12/942. Submitted to FAO by CIBA-GEIGY, Ltd., Basel, Switzerland.

Strong, M. B., Bull, M. S., Shume, G., and Kearney, E. M. 1983. Pharmacokinetic studies carried out with CGA 89317: Influence of (a) individual sheep, (b) oesophageal groove reflex and (c) formulations on the plasma levels of parent and metabolite compounds. CIBA-GEIGY Australia Ltd., R & D Technical Report 83/3/948. Submitted to FAO by CIBA-GEIGY, Ltd., Basel, Switzerland.

Strong, M. B., Adams, S. and Kearney, E. M. 1986. Plasma profiles of CGA 110752 and CGA 110753 in sheep following treatment of drench formulations of CGA 89317 prepared from alternate physical forms of the active material. CIBA-GEIGY Australia Ltd., R & D Technical Report 86/21/1063. Submitted to FAO by CIBA-GEIGY, Ltd., Basel, Switzerland.

Tournayre, J. C. 1986. Rapport d'étude de la concentration en CGA 89317 et ses métabolites (sulfoxyde et sulfone) dans le sérum d'équidés (chevaux, poneys). CIBA-GEIGY France, Report GEY/1c, December 8, 1986. Submitted to FAO by CIBA-GEIGY, Ltd., Basel, Switzerland.

FURAZOLIDONE

IDENTITY

Chemical name: 3-[[(5-nitro-2-furanyl)methylene]-amino]-2-oxazolidinone

CAS number: 67-45-8

Structural formula:

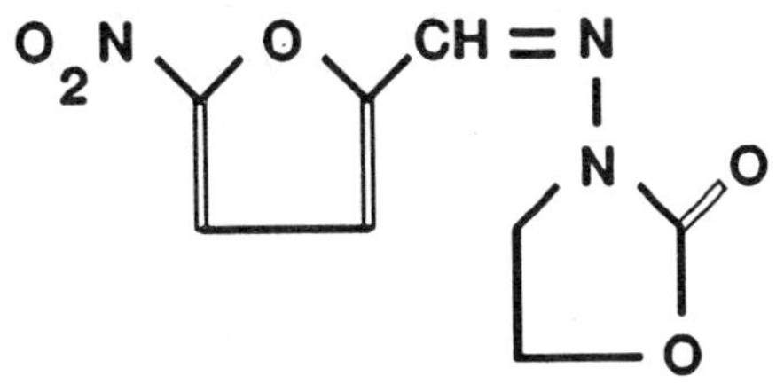

Molecular formula: $C_8H_7N_3O_5$

Molecular weight: 225.2

OTHER INFORMATION ON IDENTITY AND PROPERTIES

Pure active ingredient: Furazolidone

Appearance: Yellow crystalline powder

Melting point: 275°C

Solubility:
Slightly soluble in water, c. 40 mg per L.
Slightly soluble in 95% ethanol, c. 90 mg per L
Slightly soluble in chloroform, c. 200 mg per L.
Sparingly soluble in dimethylformamide
Insoluble in ether

UV maxima: 262 nm and 356 nm

Stability: Unstable in alkali and light

RESIDUES IN FOOD AND THEIR EVALUATION

CONDITIONS OF USE

The nitrofurans are most commonly administered by the oral route in both animal and human medicine. Solutions, suspensions, capsules, tablets, powders for reconstitution and veterinary feed premixes are available. Topical ointments, aerosol powders, soluble dressings, urethral and vaginal suppositories, and ophthalmic, nasal and ear solutions have also been developed to accommodate other routes of administration.

Furazolidone is a broad spectrum antibiotic and also has some antiprotozoal activity. It is often used as a second line antibiotic particulary when bacteria are found to be resistant to other first line antibiotics. It is used a feed additive for pigs and poultry both therapeutically and as a prophylactic for gastrointestinal and respiratory disorders.

The length of administration of the drug varies between very short periods for some therapeutic uses and almost continuous administration as an in-feed additive.

METABOLISM

Pharmacokinetics

In rats 50% of the administered dose was absorbed from the gastrointestinal tract and is mainly excreted in the urine. In pigs in a 48 hour period after oral dosing with formyl-labelled ^{14}C-Furazolidone up to 70% of the label is excreted in the urine with 12-19% excreted in the faeces and c. 3% in the expired air. The excretion in the faeces may be due to metabolism in the GI tract or entero-hepatic recirculation of the metabolites. Vroomen et al. (1986a) fed pigs with methylene-labelled ^{14}C-furazolidone and found 61% of the label excreted in the urine and 18% in the faeces over the treatment period and a 14 day withdrawal period. No label was found in the expired air. In piglets a plasma half-life of about 0.45 hours was calculated. (Yamamoto et al., 1978).

Metabolism in Food Animals.

The metabolism of the nitrofurans is extensive and complex. There is evidence of rapid degradation of the molecule yielding numerous and mostly unidentified polar metabolites. Some of the metabolites have been identified in pig urine or following *in vitro* studies with liver microsomes Vroomen, 1886). An unknown fraction of the metabolites enter the endogenous pool. There is also a substantial fraction of unidentified residues which are in the bound fraction. So far it is not possible to select either the parent drug nor any metabolite as a marker substance to indicate the level of total residues.

Dried liver, liver isolate and urine samples from treated pigs have been tested for mutagenic potential. None exhibited genetic activity in the Ames *Salmonella*/microsomal mutagenesis assay (Jaganath and Brusick, 1981).

A major route of metabolism in pigs and poultry is via the reduction of the 5-nitro group. The sponsors indicate that aerobic metabolism would predominate in the live animal and that further rapid metabolism occurs post-mortem and at low temperatures (-30°C). This would be mostly anaerobic metabolism. In a pig study Furazolidone was labelled with ^{15}N in the 5-nitro position and the urine examined. Only one minor component was identified with the ^{15}N still attached to the furan ring, suggesting that the nitro-group is removed before excretion into the urine.

By contrast more of the nitrogen in the 5-nitro group is identified in the residues in rat and rabbit urine and in rat tissues. The open chain cyano-derivative is the major metabolite in rats and is also formed during incubation studies with pig liver microsomes. (Vroomen et al., 1987) or pig hepatocytes (Hoogenboom, 1991). However it is a very minor metabolite *in vivo* in pigs as it appears to be rapidly metabolised to polar metabolites.

α-Ketoglutaric acid is a metabolite in rat urine and it might occur in pigs and poultry as an intermediate for endogenous incorporation of residues.

The bound residues in pig tissues at 0, 14, 21 and 45 days withdrawal time contain measurable amounts of the 3-amino-2-oxazolidone (3AZO) side chain. This compound is released after mild acid hydrolysis by cleavage of the azomethine bond. The amount of 3-amino-2-oxazolidone as a percentage of the bound residues in pig liver lies between 15% and 25%.

The metabolites identified in *in vivo* studies are shown on the next page.

Urinary Metabolites of Furazolidone

SPECIES

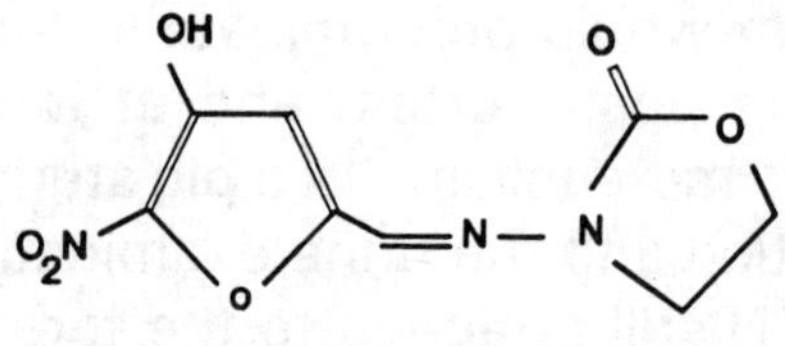

pig, chicken, rat, rabbit, dog, human

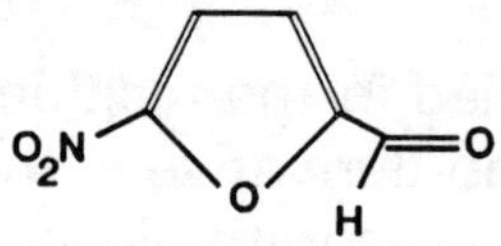

rat, pig

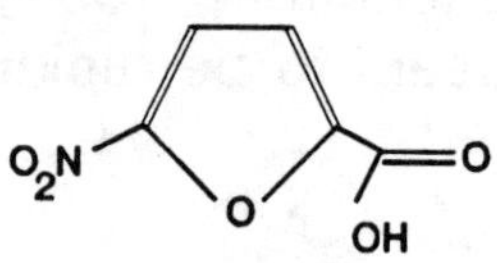

pig

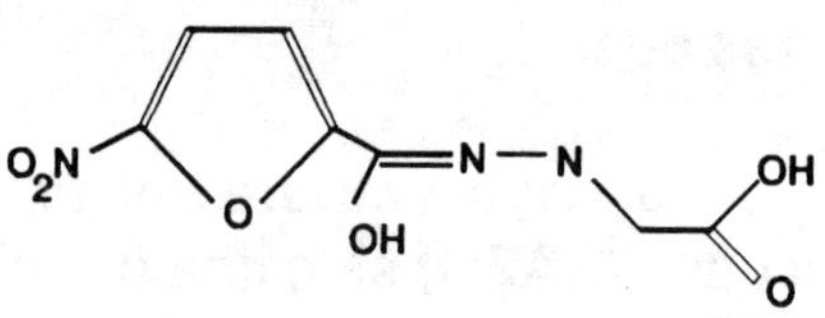

pig

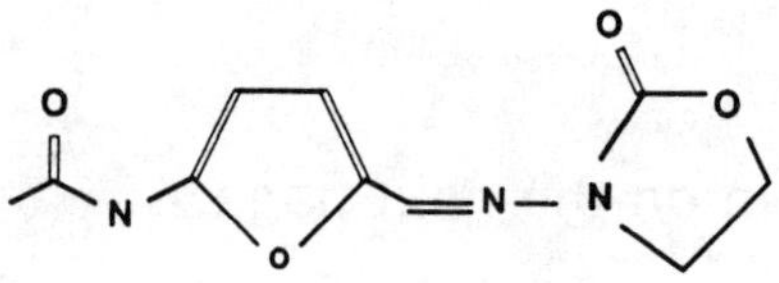

pig, rat

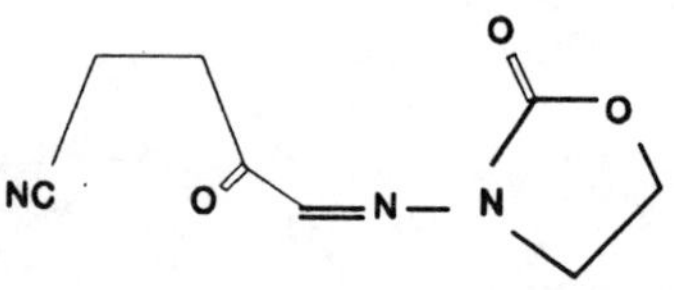

pig, rat, rabbit

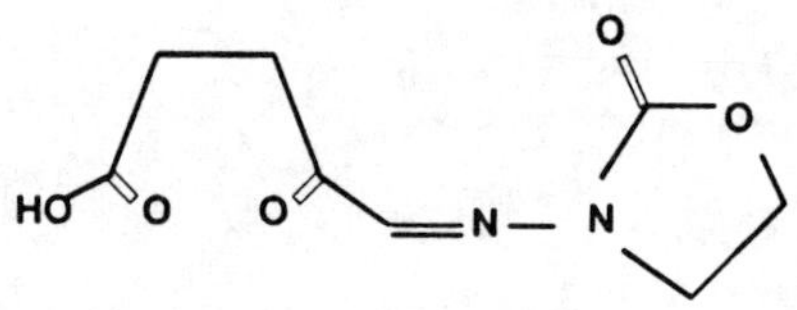

rat

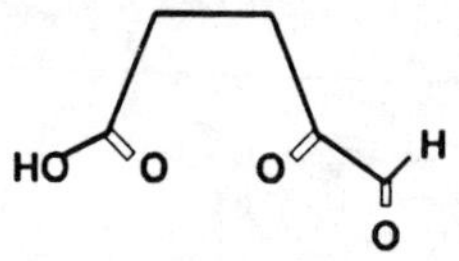

rat

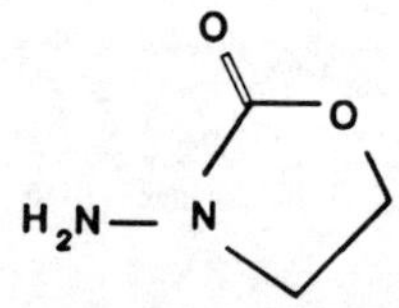

pig (after reduction of bound residues in liver and possibly formed in GI tract)

TISSUE RESIDUE DEPLETION STUDIES

Radiolabeled Residue Depletion Studies

The studies were carried out using ^{14}C-furazolidone labelled in either the formyl or methylene groups.

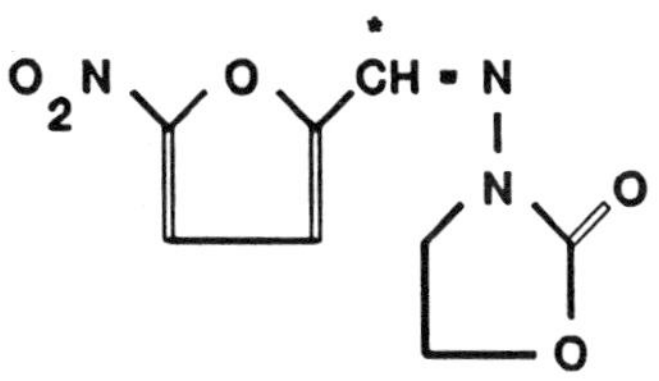

formyl label(*)

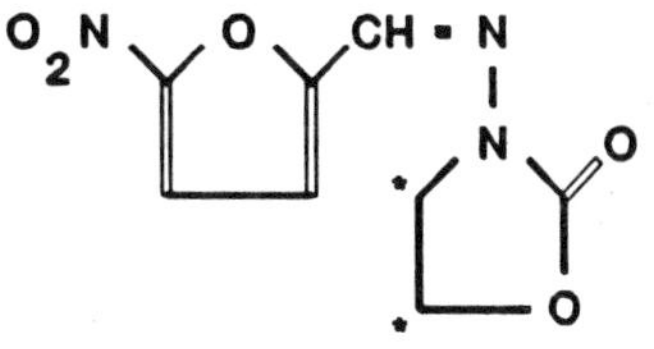

methylene label(*)

Pigs

Several radiometric studies were done in pigs. The common results were;

(i) Residues of parent drug were extremely low or absent.
(ii) Most of the residues were polar metabolites.
(iii) A significant portion of the residues were nonextractable.

Two male pigs (5.9 kg) were administered 75 mg ^{14}C-Furazolidone (formyl label) in two doses per day via a stomach tube as equivalent to 300 mg per kg in feed for 10 days or equivalent to 12 mg per kg live weight per day. Tissues were collected in one pig at 2 hours after the last dose and from the other pig 14 days after dosing. The mean levels of radioactivity (total residues) expressed as mg per kg (ppm) equivalents of Furazolidone are shown in table 1. Between 40 and 90% of the total residues can be extracted with water as polar metabolites and most of the remaining residues are nonextractable bound residues (Vroomen et al, 1986a).

Table 1. Total residues of ^{14}C-Furazolidone in pigs

Tissue	Total residue (ppm) 2 hours	Total residue (ppm) 14 days
Skin	7.3 - 9.1	2.9 - 3.5
Subcut fat	6.0	4.3
Liver	32.9 (4.8)	3.1 (0.8)
Kidney	30.1 (2.9)	3.0 (0.9)
Muscles	5.7 - 7.2 (2.3)	2.0 - 2.1 (1.2)
Lung	10.9	2.3
Heart	8.3	1.9
Testes	11.5	2.3
Bile	81.1	1.1

The values in parenthesis are the concentrations of the nonextractable portion of the residues which remain after extraction with polar and non-polar solvents and 1M urea.

The samples of muscle, fat, kidney and liver were analyzed by GC-EC and shown to contain no detectable parent drug (limit of detection; 2 μg per kg).

In two studies by Craine (1977, 1978) two female pigs weighing 5.4 kg and 7.7 kg, were fed for five days 5 mg per kg body weight of ^{14}C-furazolidone labelled in either the formyl or methylene position. The pigs were slaughtered 1 day after the last dose and the total residues, expressed as mg per kg parent drug equivalents, are shown in table 2. In another study (Tennent and Ray, 1971) a male pig weighing 26 kg was dosed with 300 mg per kg in feed for 21 days and 1.25 mg ^{14}C-Furazolidone (formyl label) on the last day. The pig was slaughtered 2 days after the last dose and the results for total residues are also shown in table 2.

Table 2. Total residues in pigs as mg per kg (ppm) parent drug equivalents

Study (Label) TISSUE	Craine 1978 (formyl) 1 day	Craine 1978 (methylene) 1 day	Tennent & Ray (formyl) 2 days
Muscle	1.00	1.02	4.5
Liver	5.15	7.80	21
Kidney	3.30	4.33	30
Fat	NA	NA	1.95

In the most recent study (Sponsor, 1991) pigs were fed ^{14}C-Furazolidone at a dose equivalent to 300 mg per kg feed for 14 days and slaughtered at 0, 21 and 45 days withdrawal time. The total residues and the residues containing the 3-amino-2-oxazolidone ring were measured. The results are shown in table 3.

Table 3. Total residues and 3-amino-2-oxazolidone in mg per kg in pig tissues

WT (days)	Liver Total	Liver AOZ	Kidney Total	Kidney AOZ	Muscle Total	Muscle AOZ
0	42.1	3.71 (8.8%)	34.7	2.10 (6.1%)	12.2	1.40 (11.5%)
0	40.0	3.08 (7.7%)	34.0	1.71 (5.0%)	14.1	1.18 (8.4%)
21	3.7	0.268 (7.2%)	2.8	0.084 (3.0%)	2.7	0.135 (5.0%)
21	5.0	0.227 (4.5%)	3.9	0.115 (2.9%)	3.8	0.085 (2.2%)
45	1.9	0.085 (4.5%)	1.6	0.035 (2.2%)	2.0	0.050 (2.5%)
45	2.4	0.075 (3.1%)	2.4	0.028 (1.2%)	2.8	0.074 (2.6%)

AOZ is 3-amino-2-oxazolidone; the figures in parenthesis are the percentage of 3-amino-2-oxazolidone of the total residues.

Chickens

Chickens were fed 220 mg ^{14}C-Furazolidone (methylene label) per kg feed for 4 days. The chickens were slaughtered and the total residues determined; the results are in table 4. Chickens were also slaughtered during a 21 day period of radiolabeled drug administration and tissue residues determined. The residues reached a maximum after eight days of Furazolidone administration and then plateaued. (Buzard et al., 1961)

Table 4. Total residues in chickens expressed as mg per kg (ppm) parent drug

WT (days)	Muscles	Liver	Kidney	Fat
0	3.40-6.08	18.6/21.1	22.1/20.8	3.53
1.5	1.58-1.89	20.8/22.1	4.06	1.11
3	0.73-1.16	3.34/3.64	2.31/2.82	1.09/1.16
5	0.70-0.87	2.32	1.39	NA
8	0.54-0.68	1.08	0.90	1.23
11	0.44-0.48	0.87	0.58	1.46

The values for muscle are the range for the residues in three different muscles determined in two chickens per time point. All other value are for individual samples.

Hens were fed ^{14}C-Furazolidone labelled in the formyl group at three levels (25, 100 and 200 mg per kg feed) for 14 days. Tissues were collected at 0, 3 and 5 days withdrawal and analyzed for Furazolidone by reverse isotope dilution. One of two samples of skin with fat at 0 days withdrawal time from hens fed 200 mg per kg contained 13 μg per kg Furazolidone. None of the other tissues exceeded 10 μg per kg the lower limit of detection of the method. No other metabolites were investigated. (Heotis et al;1969, Nº185)

Cattle

There are no radiometric studies.

OTHER RESIDUE DEPLETION STUDIES

Pigs

After medicated feed (300 mg per kg) was fed to pigs for eight days residues of Furazolidone as parent drug declined from 61 μg per kg at 0.5 hours withdrawal time to control values in less than 6.5 hours after drug withdrawal. The study also showed that the residues degraded in deep frozen tissue but not in plasma samples (Carignan et al., 1990).

Pigs were fed 300 mg Furazolidone per kg of feed for 24 days. Residues of the parent drug and metabolites with the 5-nitro-furan ring structure in tact were found in muscle (11 μg per kg), kidney (<2 to 3.1 μg per kg), skin (8.7 μg per kg) at zero withdrawal time and not detected in liver or fat tissues; the skin of 1 of 3 pigs also contained residues at 1 day withdrawal time (Hobson, 1976).

Fourteen pigs were fed 14 mg Furazolidone per kg body weight for 7 days. The pigs were slaughtered at 0, 1, 2, 4, 5, 7, 14, 21 and 28 days after drug withdrawal. Piglets were fed 6 mg Furazolidone per kg body weight for 4 days and then slaughtered at 0, 1, 2, 4, 5 and 7 days after dosing. No residues of Furazolidone (limit of detection 1 μg per kg) were found in muscle, liver, kidney, fat or heart (Shaw, 1990).

Cattle

The half life of the parent drug is short and the drug rapidly degrades at temperatures down to -30°C in tissues of calves (Nouws and Laurensen, 1990).

Six calves were dosed orally with 16 mg Furazolidone per kg body weight per day for five days. The calves were sacrificed at 0, 1, 2, 4, 5 and 7 days after the last dose. Residues of Furazolidone in muscle tissue were analyzed by HPLC. Residues of Furazolidone (33 μg per kg) were found in muscle immediately after withdrawal (day 0) of the drug although these had disappeared after storage at -20°C for three weeks (Shaw, 1990). Residues were not detected at other withdrawal times.

Female calves were fed 10 or 20 mg Furazolidone per kg body per day for ? days. They were slaughtered 17 days after the last dose. No residues were detected in muscle, liver, kidney or fat (Kalim, 1990).

Poultry

No residues of Furazolidone were found in tissues of turkeys and chickens fed 400 mg per kg feed for 14 days and 200 mg per kg feed for 7 weeks respectively except in the skin of chickens, (Winterlin et al, 1982, 1984). Residues of Furazolidone are found in eggs for up to five days after drug withdrawal (Petz, 1984) and in hen tissues in the order 3-13 μg per kg following oral doses of 10 mg per kg body weight per day for 1-10 days (Yadava et al 1986).

Day old chicks were administered 55 mg Furazolidone per kg feed for 42 days and residues of 5-nitro-furan compounds were detected in liver (0.5-1.1 μg per kg) and muscle (up to 2.9 μg per kg) at zero withdrawal time but no residues were detected at 2 days after withwrawal (Parks and Kubena, 1990).

Chickens were fed 440 mg Furazolidone per kg feed for 10 days. The chickens were killed at 0, 1, 2, 4, 5 and 7 days after dosing. The concentration of residues of Furazolidone in muscle were;

Days after dosing	0	1	2	3	4	5 & 7
Furazolidone (μg/kg)	0.8	1.8	0.5	1.0	2.4	ND

ND is not detected. Data from Shaw (1990).

<u>Other species</u>

Residues have also been reported in tissues of goats (Mustafa et al, 1985) and trout (Schmidt and Buning-Pfaue, 1985).

For the fluids, residues of Furazolidone were found in the urine of chickens (Craine and Ray, 1972) and goats and also in milk of goats (Pandey et al., 1980).

Bound Residues

There is evidence that a large portion of the total residues are in the bound fraction and the percentage although not the absolute amount of bound residues increases with the withdrawal time (see table 1).

Some further evidence (see table 5) of the amounts of free and bound residues became available in April 1992 from a recently completed bioavailability study. The pig muscle and liver samples are the same as those reported in table 3. The non-extractable radioactive residues were measured in the fraction remaining after extraction of the tissues with solvents (1. methanol : water, 1:1 v/v, ; 2. methanol; 3. ether; 4. ethyl acetate). The majority of the residues are in the bound fraction.

Table 5. Extractable (Free) and Bound residues in pig liver and muscle

Tissue	WT (days)	Total mg/kg	Free mg/kg	Bound mg/kg
Liver	0	41	18	23
Liver	45	2.15	0.18	1.97
Muscle	45	2.4	0.33	2.07

The bound residues can be divided into three types;

(i) Residues as metabolites which are of toxicological concern
(ii) Residues as metabolites which are of no toxicological concern
(iii) Residues which have entered the metabolic pool and become endogenously incorporated into cellular material and compounds

The bound residues in group (i) are the most important from a toxicology view, however the residues have not been identified or shown to be separate from those in group (ii). There is some evidence of minor mutagenic substances in rat urine and Hoogenboom (1991) showed that he could release 15-25% of the bound residues in pig liver as compounds with the 3-amino-2-oxazolidone side chain. 60% of the total residues in <u>*in vitro*</u> studies with pig hepatocytes also contained this side chain Hoogenboom 1991).

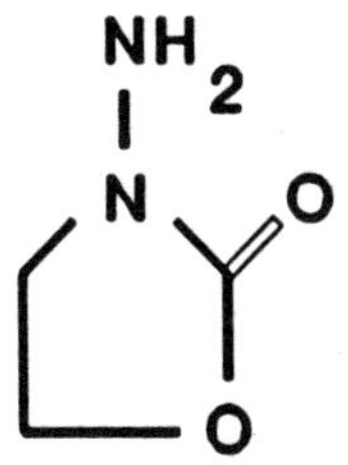

3-amino-2-oxazolidone

Metabolites with the 5-nitrofuran moiety intact may be present but have not been identified.

The fraction entering the endogenous pool is not known. In rats and chicks fed ^{14}C-Furazolidone there was expiration of radiolabeled CO_2 suggesting metabolism into the metabolic pool (via α-keto-glutarate). 3% of the label was expired in pigs administered ^{14}C-Furazolidone labelled in the formyl group but no radioactivity was expired if the label was in the methylene group. This might suggest that the oxazolidone ring does not become metabolised to form precursors for endogenous incorporation.

In summary; there is abundant evidence of bound residues and it might be assumed that much of the residue is of no toxicological concern, however more evidence is needed to apportion what fraction of the bound is toxic.

Bioavailability

The bioavailability of the bound residues was measured by refeeding lyophilized pig tissues to rats and measuring the amount of radioactivity absorbed and excreted (Sponsor study, HRC/SMI 125/911478, submitted in uncorrected final draft, April, 1992).

The incurred pig liver and muscle tissues were the same as those reported in tables 3 and 5. The bioavailability of free ^{14}C-furazolidone was also measured in three experiments in which ^{14}C-furazolidone was;

(i) Added direct to stomach of rat
(ii) Included in pelleted feed
(iii) Included as spike in lyophilised control (blank) liver and muscle.

The results are summarised in tables 6 and 7.

Table 6. Bioavailability of free ^{14}C-furazolidone

^{14}C-Furazolidone Administration	Vehicle	% absorbed
Direct to stomach	solvent	87
in pelleted feed	feed	90
Spike at 300 mg/kg	liver	73
Spike at 300 mg/kg	muscle	96

Table 7. Bioavailability of Residues in pig liver and muscle

Incurred Tissue	Residue Type	WT (days)	% absorbed	% total absorbed
Liver	Total	0	40	40
Liver	Total	45	19	19
Muscle	Total	0	37	37
Muscle	Total	45	41	41
Liver	Bound	0	31	17.4
Liver	Bound	45	16	14.7
Muscle	Bound	45	37	31.8

Combining the residue data in table 5 with the data in table 7, the amount of bioavailable residue in the free and bound fraction is calculated and shown in table 8.

Table 8. Bioavailability of free and bound residues in pig liver and muscle

Tissue	WT (days)	Free mg/kg	**Bioavailable** Free mg/kg	Bound mg/kg	**Bioavailable** Bound mg/kg
Liver	0	18	10.4	23	7.15
Liver	45	0.18	0.09	1.971	0.32
Muscle	45	0.33	0.22	2.07	0.77

The results indicate two main points;

1. The free residues are not all bioavailable, even for the parent drug added direct to the stomach.
2. The fraction of bound residues which are bioavailable is in the range 16% to 37%. In liver tissue this is equivalent to 7.15 mg/kg at day 0 withdrawal time and 0.32 mg/kg at day 45. In muscle the only measurements were made at 45 days withdrawal time and 0.77 mg/kg of bound residues are bioavailable.

In another study bioavailability was similary determined by feeding rats the nonextractable fraction of muscle tissues of piglets fed radiolabeled furazolidone for 10 days and slaughtered at zero withdrawal time. Approximately 41% of the residues were bioavailable (Vroomen et al, 1990).

Since the toxicology of the bioavailable bound residues is not known they will need to be equated with parent drug.

METHODS OF ANALYSIS FOR RESIDUES IN TISSUES

So far there is no recognised marker substance since the parent drug is rarely found as a residue. Nevertheless many countries regulate the drug by monitoring for Furazolidone. Investigations are proceeding into the possible conversion of residues into the 3-amino-2-oxazolidone molecule and it's use as a marker residue (Hoogenboom, 1991). Residues of 3-amino-2-oxazolidone were detected in pig liver at up to 45 days withdrawal time. The method for measuring 3-amino-2-oxazolidone has the following steps;

- Homogenate of liver containing 5-10 mg protein
- Incubate with 0.1*N* HCl and 0.5mM 2-nitro benzaldehyde for 20 hours at 37°C
- Extract with ethyl acetate
- Measure on HPLC with UV detection at 275 nm

This method is still in the development stage (Hoogenboom, 1991).

There are many, both old and recent, methods which are satisfactory for the routine screening or monitoring of residues of the parent drug. A review of methods for nitrofurans up to 1984 is provided by Kalim (1985). The methods are all based on a form of chromatography with various end-point detection systems. The most widely used methods have many of the following steps;

Homogenise tissue → Solvent extraction with or without a gel → cartridge column chromatography → HPLC with UV, diodearray or electrochemical detection or GC with electron capture detection.

The methods have limits of determination of c. 0.2 to 2 μg per kg and are well validated for accuracy and precision. (e.g. Laurenson & Nouws, 1989; Aerts et al, 1990; Petz, 1982, 1983; Vroomen et al., 1986; Winterlin et al, 1981).

APPRAISAL

The metabolism and residue pattern of Furazolidone is not unlike that of the nitroimidazoles reviewed at the 34th meeting. The drug is well absorbed, extensively metabolised and excreted mainly in the urine. The parent drug has a short half life both *in vivo* and in post-mortem tissues, it is either not found as a residue or at very low concentrations at zero withdrawal time. The parent drug is occasionally found at slightly longer withdrawal times, although the results from the numerous studies are sometimes confused by treatment and assay method.

The most important point for discussion is the nature of the residues. The total residues are in the mg per kg range of which ≤1000th are parent drug. Most of the residues are polar compounds in either the free or bound form. Information is lacking on either the chemical nature or the toxicity of the majority of the residues although there is some indication that the residues in swine liver and urine do not possess genetic activity in the Ames Salmonella/microsomal mutagenesis assay. The half life of the parent drug is very short but the half-life of the total residues is very long because many of the metabolites are either bound or enter the endogenous pool.

Many metabolites resulting from *in vitro* studies in rats and pigs have been identified or at least postulated . The 5-nitro group is rapidly reduced in microsome preparations. Also both the furan and azolidone rings may be opened and cyano or keto end groups are among the possibilities. In *in vivo* studies there is evidence of extensive reduction of the 5-nitro group which continues in the post-mortem tissues. The nitrogen in the 5-nitro group and still attached to the furan ring is found in a significant fraction of the residues both excreted by the rat and rabbit and also in the incubation mixtures of the rat, chicken and pig microsomes, but it is only a very minor fraction of the residues in pigs. The ring structure of the oxazolidone is still present in some of the residues in pig tissues.

There is evidence for incorporation of the residues into the endogenous pool in rats, chickens and pigs. The fractions entering the endogenous pool are not known.

The percentage of residues in the bound fraction increases with withdrawal time. In pigs the 3-amino-2-oxazolidone group can be released from at least 15-25% of the bound residues in liver tissue. The bound residues constitute a significant amount (c. 1 mg per kg or higher) of the residues.

The bioavailability studies show that

1. The free residues are only 52% to 67% bioavailable, even the parent drug added direct to the stomach of rats was only 87% absorbed.

2. The fraction of bound residues which are bioavailable is in the range 16% to 37%. In liver tissue this is equivalent to 10 mg/kg at day 0 withdrawal time and 0.32 mg/kg at day 45. In muscle the only measuremnets were made at 45 days withdrawal time and 0.77 mg/kg of bound residues are bioavailable.

The toxicology of the bound residues is not known. In the absence of this information the potency of the bound residues will need to be considered.

Information is submitted on residues from cold studies in which only residues of the parent drug or the 5-nitro-furfurylaldehyde (after derivatisation) were measured. Residues were sometimes detected at short withdrawal times in pigs, poultry, goats and trout.

There are several well validated analytical methods for measuring and regulating residues of the parent drug. A technical problem is caused by the rapid degradation of Furazolidone in post-mortem tissues at temperatures down to -30°C.

Recent studies indicate that the measurement of residues of 3-amino-2-oxazolidone may offer a possible marker residue for pigs. Residues of this compound are detectable for at least a 45 day withdrawal period.

REFERENCES

Aerts, M.M.L., Beek, W.M.J and Brinkman, U.A.Th. 1990. On-line combination of dialysis and column switching chromatography as a fully automated sample preparation technique for biological samples. Determination of nitrofuran residues in edible products. J.Chrom., 500, 453-468.

Buzard, J.A, Heotis, J.P. and Williams, C.W. 1961. Chick distribution studies with C14-(formyl)-NF-180. Interim Report Nº360.3, Sponsor submission.

Carignan, G., MacIntosh, A.I. and Sved, S. 1990. An assay for furazolidone residues by liquid chromatography with electrochemical detection applicable to depletion studies in pigs. J.Agric.Food Chem., **38**, 716-720.

Craine, E.M. 1978b. Research reports. The extraction and analysis of ^{14}C residues occurring in the tissues of pigs treated with Furazolidone-^{14}C. Research Report NºEMC 78:15.

Craine, E.M. and Ray, W.H. 1972. Metabolites of Furazolidone in urine of chickens. J. Pharm. Sci., **61**, 1495-1497.

Craine, E.M. 1977 and 1978a. Research reports. The disposition of Furazolidone-^{14}C to the urine and tissues of pigs. Research Reports NºEMC 77:10 (1977) and EMC 78:12 (1978a)

Heotis,J.P., Rose, G, Olivard, J. and Teelin, R. 1969. NF-180 residues in chicken tissues. Report Nº185, Sponsor submission.

Hobson, D.L. 1976. Tissuer residue studies of swine receiving 300 grams Furazolidone per ton of feed for 24 days. Research report Nº DLH 76:51 submitted by sponsor.

Hoogenboom, L.A.P. 1991. Doctoral Thesis, The use of pig hepatocytes for biotranformation and toxicity studies. RIKILT, Wageningen, Holland.

HRC/SMI 1992. The bioavailability in rats of tissue residues from swine administered ^{14}C-furazolidone for 14 days and subjected to 0-day, 21-day and 45-day withdrawal periods. Report Nº, 125/911478 submitted as uncorrected final draft by sponsors.

Jaganath, D.R. and Brusick, D.J. 1981. Toxicity of residues. Sponsors submission, Ref.Nº 228-234.

Kalim, H. 1985. Detection of Furazolidone residues in tissues and body fluids of calves and pigs by HPLC. DVM Thesis, University of Munich.

Laurenson, J.J. & Nouws, J.F.M. 1989. Simultaneous determination of nitrofuran derivatives in various animal substrates by HPLC. J.Chrom., **472**, 321-326.

Mustafa, A.I., Ali, B.H. and Hassan, T. 1985. Semen characteristics in Furazolidone-treated goats. Reprod. Nutr. Develop., **27(1A)**, 89-94.

Nouws, J.F.M. and Laurenson, J.J. 1990. Postmortal degradation of furazolidone and furaltadone in edible tissues of calves. The Vet. Quart., **12**, 56-59.

Pandey, S.N., Banerjee, N.C. and Singh. 1980. Comparative study of nitrofurantoin and Furazolidone in caprine plasma and milk. Indian J. Pharmacol., 12, 193-196.

Parks, O.W. and Kubena, L.F. 1990. Liquid chromatography-electrochemical detection of Furazolidone and metabolites in extracts of incurred tissues. J.A.O.A.C., **73**, 526-528.

Petz, M. 1983. HPLC method for the determination of residual chloramphenicol, Furazolidone and five sulphonamides in eggs, meat and milk. Z. Lebensm. Unters Forsch., **176**, 289-293.

Petz, M. 1984. Rückstande im Ei nach Behandlung von Legehennen mit Chloramphenicol und Furazolidone. Arch. für Lebensmittelhygiene, **35**, 49-72.

Petz, M. 1982. Method for determination of furazolidone and four other nitrofurans in eggs, meat and milk by HPLC. Dtsch. Lebensm-Rundsch., **78**, 396-401.

Schmidt, Th. and Büning-Pfaue, H. 1985. Rückstandverhalten von Arzneistoffen in der Intensivhaltung von Nutzfishen. Deutsch. Lebensm.-Rundsch., **81**, 239-243.

Shaw, I.C. 1990. Furazolidone: Pharmacokinetics and residues in calves, chickens and pigs (adult and piglet) 2 volumes, CVL, Weybridge.

Tennent, D.M. and Ray, W.H. 1971. Metabolism of Furazolidone in swine (35994) Proc. Exp. Biol. Med., **138**, 808-810.

Vroomen L.H.M. 1986. Doctoral Thesis "In vivo and in vitro metabolic studies of furazolidone." RIKILT, Wageningen.

Vroomen, L.H.M., Van Ohmen, B. and Van Bladern, P.J. 1987. Quantitative studies of the metabolism of furazolidone by rat liver microsomes. Toxic. in Vitro, 1, 97-104.

Vroomen, L.H.M., Berghmans, M.C.J., Van Bladeren, P.J., Groten, J.P., Wissink, A.C.J. and Kuiper, H.A. 1988 and 1990. Bound residues of furazolidone. A potential hazard for the consumer. Proc. Eur. A.V.P.T. (1988) Eds., F. Simon, P. Lees and G. Semjen, (1990).

Vroomen, L.H.S., Berghmans, M.C.J. Van Leeuwen, P., Van der Struijs, T.D.B, De Vries, H.U. and Kuiper, H.A. 1986a. Kinetics of ^{14}-C-furazolidone in piglets upon oral administration during 10 days and its interaction with tissue macromolecules. Food Additives & Contamin., **3**, 331-346.

Vroomen, L.H.S., Berghmans, M.C.J. and Van der Struijs. T.D.B. 1986b. Determination of furazolidone in swine plasma, muscle, liver, kidney fat and urine based on HPLC separation after solid-phase extraction on Extrelut® 1. J.Chromatog., **362**, 141-145.

Winterlin, W., Mourer, C., Hall, G., Kratzer, F., Ogasawara, F., Brown, C. McClaughlin, H. Crew, M and Weaver, G. 1982. Furazolidone in turkey tissues following a 14-day feeding trial. Poultry Science, **61**, **1113-1117**.

Winterlin, W., Hall, G., and Mourer, C. 1981. Drug residues in animal tissues: Ultra-trace determination of furazolidone in turkey tissues by liquid partitioning and HPLC. J.A.O.A.C., **64**, 1055-1059.

Winterlin, W., Mourer, C., Hall, G., Kratzer, Weaver, G., Tribble, L.F. and Kim, S.M. 1984. Furazolidone residues in chicken and swine tissues after feeding trials. J. Environ. Sci and Health, **B19**, 209-224.

Yadava, K.P., Pandey, S.N. and Banerjee, N.C. 1986. Pharmacokinetics of furazolidone in White Leghorn *Gallus domesticus*. Indian vet. J., **63**, **460-466**.

Yamamoto, H., Yamaoka, R. and Kohanawa, M. 1978. Residue of furazolidone in swine administered orally. Ann. Rep. Nat. Vet. Assay Lab., **15**, 57-61.

NITROFURAZONE

IDENTITY

Chemical name: 2-[(5-nitro-2-furanyl)methylene]-hydrazinecarboxamide or 5-nitro-2-furaldehyde semicarbazone

CAS number: 59-87-0

Structural formula:

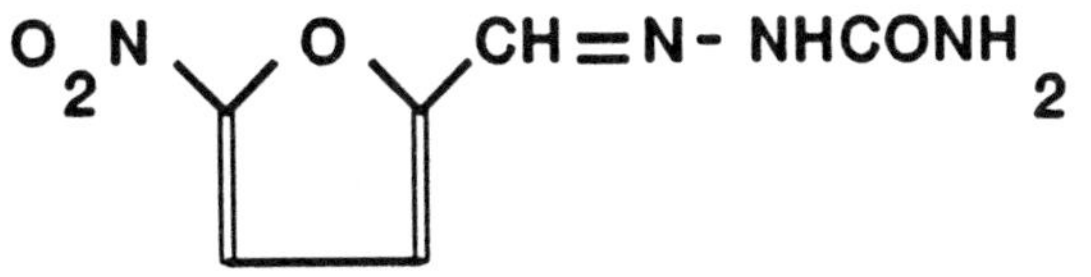

Molecular formula: $C_6H_6N_4O_4$

Molecular weight: 198.14

OTHER INFORMATION ON IDENTITY AND PROPERTIES

Pure active ingredient: Nitrofurazone

Appearance: Yellow needles or crystalline powder

Melting point: 236-240°C (decomposes)

Solubility: Slightly soluble in water, c. 240 mg per L.
Slightly soluble in 95% ethanol, c.1.69 g per L
Soluble in dimethylformamide, 1 g in 15 mL
Soluble in alkaline solutions
Not soluble in chloroform, ether or benzene

UV maxima: 264 nm and 367 nm

Stability: Unstable in light

RESIDUES IN FOOD AND THEIR EVALUATION

CONDITIONS OF USE

The nitrofurans are most commonly administered by the oral route in both animal and human medicine. Solutions, suspensions, capsules, tablets, powders for reconstitution and veterinary feed premixes are available. Topical ointments, aerosol powders, soluble dressings, urethral and vaginal suppositories, and ophthalmic, nasal and ear solutions have also been developed to accommodate other routes of administration.

Nitrofurazone is a broad spectrum antibiotic and also has some antiprotozoal activity. It is often used as a second line antibiotic particulary when bacteria are found to be resistant to other first line antibiotics. It is used a feed additive for pigs and poultry both therapeutically and as a prophylactic for gastrointestinal and respiratory disorders.

The length of administration of the drug varies between very short periods for some therapeutic uses and almost continuous administration as an in-feed additive.

METABOLISM

Pharmacokinetics

Pharmacokinetic studies were carried out in rats and calves. ^{14}C-Nitrofurazone (aldehyde-labelled) was administered as a single oral dose to male rats. The rats were either prefed or not fed "cold" Nitrofurazone. Rapid excretion of the radioactivity was exhibited by all the rats, with an average of 100.5% of the administered radioactivity appearing in the urine, bile, faeces and exhaled CO_2 within 48 hours. Tissue residues at 48 hours after dosing were <1 mg per kg. There were no differences in Nitrofurazone residues between rats from the two feeding regimens (Bowman, 1961).

^{14}C-Nitrofurazone was administered orally to rats. 88% of the radioactivity administered was absorbed from the gastrointestinal tract into the bile and urine. After 96 hours almost all of the radioactivity administered was excreted in the urine and faeces. Only a small amount (not stated) was excreted as parent drug (Tatsumi et al., 1971).

A single dose of nitrofurazone (14 mg per kg body weight) was administered to five preruminant calves. Peak plasma concentrations (mean 3.5 mg per L) were observed at approximately 3 hours after administration. The final elimination half-life was 5 hours. The renal clearance of the unbound drug was c. 0.42 ml/min/kg. Less than 2% of the administered dose was recovered as parent drug in the urine. (Nouws et al., 1986)

Metabolism in Food Animals

No detailed metabolism studies were available. As Nitrofurazone is a minor fraction of excreted residues in preruminant cattle and presumably other farm animals, it is certain that Nitrofurazone is extensively metabolised. One might assume that the 5-nitro group is reduced to the amine. However in the absence of radiometric studies or "cold" drug studies in food animals the only conclusion is that the parent drug is extensively metabolised to unknown metabolites.

Metabolism in Laboratory Animals

Tatsumi et al, (Sponsor Abstracts, Nº 455-459) studied the absorption, excretion and metabolism of Nitrofurazone in rats. Nitrofurazone is readily absorbed from the GI tract, extensively metabolised and rapidly excreted. In *in vivo* and *in vitro* studies the drug is metabolised in the mucosa wall of the small intestine. One identified route was the reduction of the 5-nitro group to the amine involving the enzyme, xanthine oxidase. The metabolites were less well absorbed than the parent compound.

The xanthine oxidase system in milk also reduces Nitrofurazone to the 5-amine. (Taylor et al.,1951).

After the incubation of ^{14}C-Nitrofurazone in the presence of 9,000g rat liver supernatant or xanthine oxidase-hypoxanthine, three unidentified metabolites were found by HPLC, one of which was thought to be a cysteine conjugate (Goodman et al.). Further evidence for both the aerobic and anaerobic reduction of the 5-nitro group by the xanthine oxidoreductase system in rat liver extracts is reported by Kutcher et al. (1984).

Paul et al., (1960) sugggested that Nitrofurazone is metabolised in mammalian tissues both by 5-nitro reduction and cleavage of the -CH=N- linkage and that none of the end products posessed antibacterial properties.

TISSUE RESIDUE DEPLETION STUDIES

Radiolabeled Residue Depletion Studies

No studies are available for food animals. In rats no residues were identified at the 1 mg per kg level (Bowman, 1961).

Residue Depletion Studies with Unlabeled Drug

Four pigs were fed Nitrofurazone at 0.011% inclusion in the feed for ? days. The pigs were killed at zero withdrawal time. The tissues analysed for Nitrofurazone by extracting the Nitrofurazone and measuring the UV spectra between 400-460 nm. Quantitation was made by iteration against standards at 430 nm and subtracting the blank value for untreated pigs. The residues in liver, kidney, fat, ham and loin were all <0.1 mg per kg. (SKB submission from study done 1967).

One-day-old chicks were raised to maturity on a diet fortified with 0.0055% Nitrofurazone. At 42 days of age nine chickens were sacrificed, the tissues from pairs of birds (and on single bird) were blended and residues measured by the method of Parks (1989). The results are shown in table 1. A further nine birds were sacrificed following a two day withdrawal of the drug. No residues (<0.5 μg per kg) were detected in these birds. (Parks and Kubena, 1992).

Comment: The tissues were sampled quickly and immediately frozen to temperatures <-50°C, sometimes using liquid nitrogen. Nevertheless there is no appraisal of the stability of the nitrofurazone under these conditions of storage. Laurensen and Nouws (1989) stabilised the Nitrofurazone by immediately homogenising the samples in buffer before freezing (see below).

Table 1. Residues of Nitrofurazone (μg per kg) in Chickens fed Nitrofurazone

Bird numbers	Liver	Thigh	Breast
1024, 1028	146	2.22	2.64
1033, 1040	120	2.20	1.39
1047, 1053	87	1.17	0.69
1058, 1065	148	2.30	2.72
1067	63	9.11	5.36
All (mean ± SD)	113 ± 37	3.40 ± 3.23	2.56 ± 1.78

Chickens were fed Nitrofurazone at 150 g per ton of feed for 14 days and the residues measured at 3, 4 and 5 days after drug withdrawal (Mertz, 1971). The results are shown in table 2.

Table 2. Residues Nitrofurazone (μg per kg) in chickens

Tissue	3 days WT	4 days WT	5 days WT
Liver		<2 (7)	<2 (5)
Muscle		<2 (4)	<2 (4)
Skin with fat		<2 (4)	<2 (4)
Kidney	<2 (3), 2 (1)	<2 (2)	<2 (1), 2 (1)

The number of chickens are given in parentheses.

Bound Residues/Bioavailability

No evidence was available.

METHODS OF ANALYSIS FOR RESIDUES IN TISSUES

Summary: As indicated above, Nitrofurazone was shown to be less than 2% of the total residues of the dosed animals. It is assumed that Nitrofurazone almost certainly forms a very minor proportion of the total residues in the edible tissues. Nevertheless there are numerous validated methods for measuring residues of the parent drug. Four of the methods are discussed.

A TLC method for Nitrofurazone in tissues of chickens was one of the earlier developed methods. After homogenisation, exhaustive solvent-solvent partition and chromatography on a celite:silica gel column an aliquot of the final extract was run on a TLC plate. The Nitrofurazone spot was measured at 360 nm. This method is semi-quantitative and claims a lower limit of detection of 2 μg per kg Nitrofurazone in chicken kidney. (Heotis et al, 1971).

A gas chromatography - electron capture detection (GC-ECD) method for determing Nitrofurazone in chicken tissues at the 2 μg per kg level is provided by the sponsors (Hobson, 1976). Nitrofurazone was extracted into ethyl acatate. The extract was reduced in volume and transferred with benzene and hexane. The organic solution was extracted with water. The water extract was acidified and the Nitrofurazone hydrolysed at 75°C to form the 5-nitro-2-furaldehyde (NFA). The extract was placed on a Florisil column, washed with benzene, and the NFA eluted with benzene/ethyl acetate. An aliquot was placed onto a 6 foot x 4 mm column packed with 3% DEGA on Chromosorb W at 150°C. Standards were run and the amount of NFA (as Nitrofurazone) determined by iteration.

The lower limit of detection was 2 μg per kg. The average recovery of Nitrofurazone as spikes at 2 μg per kg from tissues and the CVs for the method are shown in table 3.

Table 3. Recovery of Nitrofurazone from chicken tissues

Tissue	% Recovery of 2 μg per kg spike (n = 5)	CV (%)
skin	75	5.7
muscle	76	5.2
liver	75	4.4
kidney	74	5.6

Two of the HPLC methods are detailed below.

Laurensen and Nouws (1989) describe a method which prevents degradation of the Nitrofurazone in organic tissue and measures the residue at a 1 ug per kg level by an HPLC procedure. The fresh samples of urine, plasma and edible tissues were blended or homogenised with 1.5*M* KH_2PO_4 containing 0.2% sodium azide. They were immediately frozen and stored in the dark until assayed. During extraction the samples were protected from light. The samples were extracted with dichloromethane-ethyl acetate. The extract was evaporated to dryness and taken up in a mixture of n-hexane and phospate buffer, pH 5.0. An aliquot of the aqueous phase was injected into an HPLC system. The columns were a guard column and a separation column (Zorbax CN). The eluent was sodium acetate buffer (pH 5.0) and methanol; flow rate 1.5 ml per min at 20°C. Detection was by UV at 365 nm. Quantification was done by iteration with calibration graphs using the addition of 1 to 100 ug per kg spikes. The mean recovery values and CVs are shown in table 4.

Table 4. Recovery and Reproducibility of 1-100 µg per kg Nitrofurazone in bovine tissues

Tissue	Recovery (%)	CV (%)	Linearity
plasma	69.7	3.0	0.9999
meat	60.7	2.2	0.9998
liver	60.7	2.0	0.9998

An HPLC-ECD method for measuring residues of Nitrofurazone in chicken tissues was published by Parks (1989). The method includes extraction of tissues with chloroform-ethyl acetate-dimethyl sulfoxide (50:50:8), adsorption onto neutral alumina and subsequent elution of the residues with pH 6.0 phosphate buffer-methanol. An aliquot was injected into an HPLC system with a Supelcosil LC-18 column. The mobile phase was pH 6.0 phosphate buffer-methanol and 0.001*M* EDTA running at 1 ml per min. Quantification was done by iteration with calibration graphs using the addition of 6 to 200 ug per kg spikes at 5 to 6 concentrations. The linearity was 0.9995 and the mean recovery values and CVs are shown in table 5.

Table 5. Recovery and Reproducibility of 6-200 μg per kg Nitrofurazone in chicken tissues

Tissue	Mean Recovery (%)	CV (%)
Liver	74.0	7.7
Thigh	78.7	6.1
Breast	76.8	8.1

This method has been applied to incurred chicken tissues (see above).

APPRAISAL

There is not sufficient information to establish an MRL. The major difficulty is the complete lack of information on the nature or quantity of residues in tissues of target animals. There is no radiometric study in target animals. The metabolism is probably somewhat similar to that for furazolidone in that there is extensive metabolism to numerous metabolites many of which form bound residues. There is some evidence that the 5-nitro group is reduced to the amine by the xanthine-oxidoreductase system. Whereas the parent drug rapidly disappears as a residue, the bound residues and maybe other metabolites could have long half lives. There is a need for information on the quantity, nature and toxicity of the total residues.

Following the in-feed administration of a commercial dose of drug, residues of the parent drug were measured in tissues of chickens at zero withdrawal time. The levels were highest in liver (113 μg per kg) and lowest in muscle tissue (0.7 to 9 μg per kg). At two days withdrawal time no residues (<1 μg per kg) of parent drug were detectable. In an older study residues were found at the 2 μg per kg level in the kidneys of one chicken at 3 days withdrawal time and another bird at 5 days withdrawal time. No residues at the 0.1 mg per kg level were detected in pigs at zero withdrawal time after feeding at the 0.011% inclusion level. There are several well validated methods for measuring residues of the parent drug at the 1 to 2 μg per kg level.

REFERENCES

Bowman, J.S. 1961. A balance study of nitrofurazone-C14 (aldehyde-labeled) in male rats. Hess and Clark, Sponsor abstract paper № 52.

Goodman, D., Aufrere, M., Vore, M. and Meyers, F. Metabolism of Nitrofurazone. 61st Meeting Fed. Am. Soc. Exp. Biol. (Sponsor Abs. № 154).

Heotis, J.P., et al. 1971. Chemical method for determination of concentrations of nitrofurazone in chicken kidney at 2 parts per billion. Sponsor Paper №183.

Hobson, D.L. 1976. Gas-liquid determination of nitrofurazone in chicken tissues at two parts per billion. Res. Report. Nº 4171. Sponsor submission paper Nº195.

Kutcher, W.W. and McCalla, D.R. 1984. Aerobic reduction by rat liver xanthine dehydrogenase. Biochem. Pharm., **33**, 799-805.

Laurensen, J.J. and Nouws, J.F.M. 1989. Simultaneous determination of nitrofuran derivatives in various animal substrates by high-performance liquid chromatography. J. Chrom., **472**, 321-326.

Mertz. J.L. 1971. Tissue residue withdrawal studies for Nitrofurazone at 150 grams per ton of feed for 14 days. Norwich, New York, Norwich Pharmacal Co., Nov 8, (1971). Sponsor Abs Nº 307.

Nouws, J.F.M., Vree, T.B., Aerts, M.M.L., Degen, M. and Driessens, F. 1986. Some pharmacological data about Furaltadone and Nitrofurazone administered to preruminant calves. Food Addit. Contamin., **3**, 1331-1346.

Parks, O.W. Liquid chromatographic-electrochemical detection screening procedure for six nitro-containing drugs in chicken tissues at low ppb level. J.A.O.A.C., **72**, 567-569

Parks,O.W. and Kubena, L.F. Liquid chromatographic determination of incurred nitrofurazone residues in chicken tissues.

Tatsumi, K. Ou, T., Yoshimura, H. and Tsukamoto, H. 1971. Metabolism of Drugs. LXXIII. Metabolic fate of nitrofuran derivatives. (1); Studies on Absorption and excretion. Chem. Pharm Bull., **19**, 330-334.

Taylor, J.D., Paul, H.E. and Paul M.F. 1951. Metabolism of the nitrofurans. 223-231, (1951). Sponsor Abs. Nº 462.

BOVINE SOMATOTROPIN

IDENTITY

Chemical name:

Synonyms:	bST Bovine Growth Hormone Somagrebove (American Cyanamid) Somidobove (Elanco) Sometribove (Monsanto) Somavubove (Upjohn)
Structural formula:	Pituitary-derived bST (one of four natural variants) see Figure 1
Products:	**Amino-Terminal Substitution of Ala (191)**
Somagrebove	Met-Asp-Gln
Somidobove	Met-Phe-Pro-Leu-Asp-Asp-Asp-Asp-Lys
Sometribove	Met
Somavubove	None
Molecular formula:	$C_{976}H_{1533}N_{265}O_{286}S_8$ (Figure 1)
Molecular weight:	21,812

OTHER INFORMATION ON IDENTITY AND PROPERTIES

Pure active ingredient:

Appearance: white odorless powder

Melting point: decomposition to black precipitate

RESIDUES IN FOOD AND THEIR EVALUATION

CONDITIONS OF USE

General

Bovine Somatotropin (bST) is a genetically engineered protein hormone either identical or similar to the natural bovine pituitary product. Its primary function is to increase milk production in lactating dairy cattle.

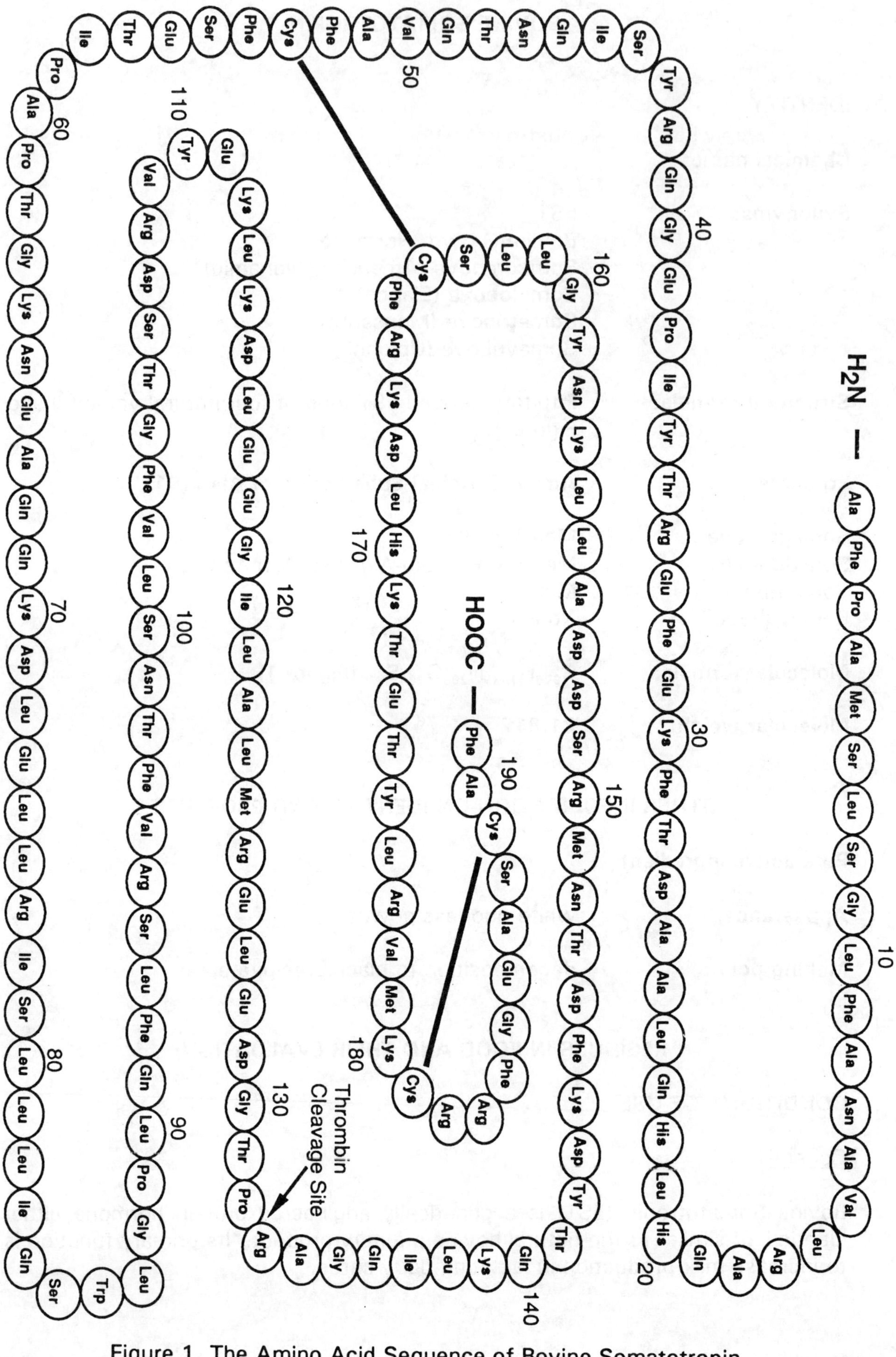

Figure 1. The Amino Acid Sequence of Bovine Somatotropin

Dosages

Bovine ST is administered to cattle via subcutaneous or intramuscular administration. A continuous application of the drug is proposed beginning approximately 50-90 days post-partum until the end of lactation. The products are administered either as a daily injectable or a 14-28 day sustained release injectable. The proposed dosage calculated on a daily basis ranges from 10-35 mg/day.

Other Residues

Since many of the effects of bST are known to be mediated by insulin-like growth factors, especially insulin-like growth factor I (IGF-I), IGF-I concentrations following bST-treatment have been determined. IGF-I is an endogenous polypeptide containing 70 amino acids (see Figure 2). Bovine and human IGF-I have the same amino acid sequence.

METABOLISM

Pharmacokinetics

Bovine ST

A study was conducted to determine if there was a difference in the pharmacokinetics of methionyl bST (sometribove) and a naturally occurring variant of bST (ALA-VAL bST) in lactating Holstein cows (Birmingham et al., 1988). A 25 mg IV bolus dose was administered to each of nine animals in a random cross-over design. Blood samples were collected over a 12-hour period and analyzed for somatotropin concentration using a homologous radioimmunoassay. A decline in serum somatotropin levels with time followed a biexponential curve described by a two-compartment open model. The pharmacokinetic estimates of both variants of bST were not significantly different ($P>0.05$). Distribution half-lives of ALA-VAL bST and sometribove averaged 0.17 and 0.12 hours, and the terminal half-lives were 0.66 and 0.52 hours, respectively. Total body clearances were 66.99 and 68.14 L/h and volumes of distribution averaged 22.83 and 18.91 L for ALA-VAL and sometribove, respectively. These results indicate that the pharmacokinetics of methionyl-sometribove are indistinguishable from a naturally occurring somatotropin variant, ALA-VAL bST.

Two studies demonstrated that treatment with recombinant bST (rbST) increased the concentration of bST in plasma. In one study (Schams et al., 1988a), fourteen Simmental dairy cows were administered 500 mg of sometribove/ injection in the form of slow-release formulation to determine its effect on peripheral blood concentrations of bST. The cows were divided into 2 groups and sometribove was administered according to a cross over design. Group A was treated 5 times (10 weeks) at two-week intervals beginning 10 weeks after parturition, and group B was given a placebo. Three weeks after this treatment period (weeks 20-23 postpartum), group B was treated for 10 weeks with bST, and group A received a placebo (weeks 24-33). Blood for hormone analysis was sampled at weeks 13, 17, 23, 27 and 31 for 24 hour periods at 30 minute intervals. Bovine ST was analyzed by RIA.

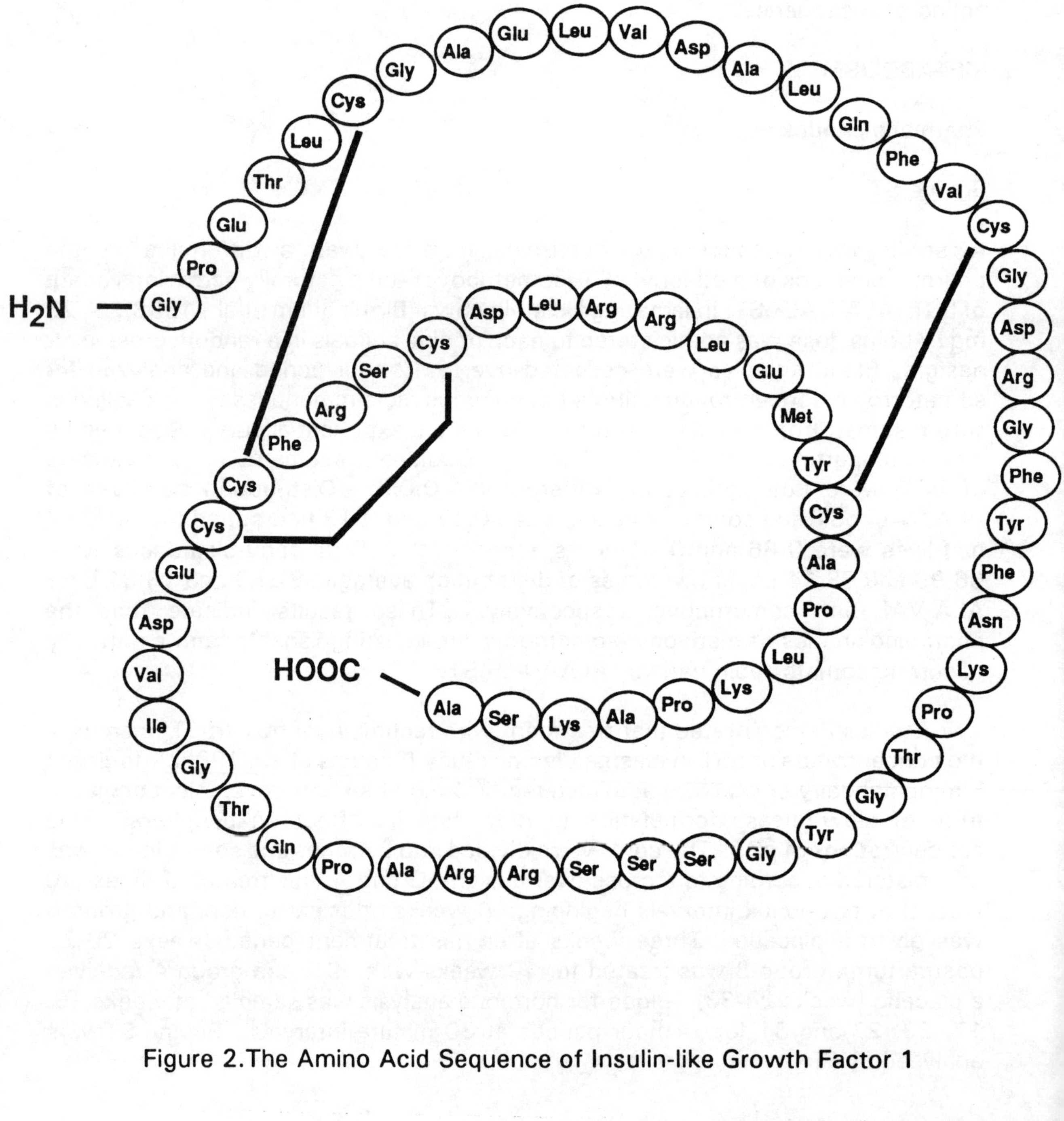

Figure 2.The Amino Acid Sequence of Insulin-like Growth Factor 1

The means of bST blood concentrations in untreated cows for the different time courses varied between 8.9 and 13.2 ng/ml. For both groups treatment with bST increased concentrations of bST about 2.4-3.2 fold to mean values of 25.8-36.1 ng/ml. There was a high variability in bST concentrations within both groups of animals.

In a series of 3 experiments, Schams and Karg (1988b) demonstrated that an increase in plasma bST levels was acheived after the animals were treated with somidobove. In the first experiment, eight cows (4 controls and 4 treated) of different breeds were used as either untreated controls or injected subcutaneously with 640 mg of somidobove. The mean blood bST levels in the controls were approximately 10 ng/ml. Bovine ST concentrations increased after the injection of bST, a maximum was reached on day 3 (42.6 ng/ml) and levels decreased to baseline by day 13. Similar results were obtained in their second experiment.

In their last experiment, forty-eight dairy cows, divided in four treatment groups, were used. The four treatment groups, containing 12 cows each, were made up of: control, high dose of somidobove (960 mg), medium dose (640 mg), and low dose (320 mg). From each animal, plasma samples were taken each week for four weeks before treatment, each week for 24 weeks after the first treatment and for four weeks after the last treatment. In general, maximum concentrations of bST were obtained during the first and second week of treatment with the high and medium dose with levels of 90 ng/ml and 50 ng/ml, respectively. For the low dose, the increase was more moderate (35 ng/ml) during the second week. Average control values were approximately 10 ng/ml. For bST, there is a tendency toward decreased plasma concentrations with an increasing number of bST treatments.

<u>IGF-I from bST-treated Cattle</u>

In a study conducted for Monsanto (Schams et al., 1988a), fourteen Simmental dairy cows were administered 500 mg of sometribove/injection in the form of a slow-release formulation to determine its effect on peripheral blood concentrations of IGF-I. The cows were divided into 2 groups and bST was administered according to a cross over design. Group A was treated 5 times (10 weeks) at two-week intervals beginning 10 weeks after parturition, and group B obtained a placebo. Three weeks after this treatment period (weeks 20-23 postpartum), group B was treated for 10 weeks with bST, and group A received a placebo (weeks 24-33). Blood for hormone analysis was sampled at weeks 13, 17, 23, 27 and 31 for 24 hour periods at 30 minute intervals. Each fifth sample was analyzed by RIA for IGF-I.

The means of IGF-I concentrations in untreated cows for the different time courses varied from 261-320 ng/ml. After bST treatment, the levels of IGF-I increased 3.1-3.9 fold to mean values of 941-1163 ng/ml. There was a high variability in IGF-I concentrations within both groups of animals.

METABOLISM IN CATTLE

Monsanto conducted studies (Rogan et al., 1988; Mehta, 1988) to isolate and characterize the bST metabolites in bovine serum. From 4 cows treated with 15 g of sometribove on day 0 and day 7, the serum was collected 7 days after injection. Bovine ST concentrations were determined by using a particle concentration sandwich fluorescent immunoassay, which measures intact bST. The results of the bST analysis of the serum were found to be 184, 208, 213, and 122 ng/ml for the individual cows.

Bovine ST and its metabolites were subjected to SDS-PAGE electrophoresis. Silver staining revealed 8-10 protein bands that ranged from 7 kd to 95 kd. Proteolytic fragments of bST produced by thrombin and intact bST were included in the electrophoresis run so that the molecular weight of any metabolites could be defined. Under reduced conditions two immunoreactive bands were seen in the isolate. The migration of the bands was identical to that of the reduced thrombin-clipped bST (7 kd and 14 kd). The intact bST band was also present but the band at 14 kd was the most intense. Under the oxidized conditions the binding pattern of the thrombin-clipped bST and the isolate were also identical. The band at 14 kd was again the most intense.

A total of 14 micrograms of bST metabolite was isolated from the 4 cows, which allowed for amino acid sequencing. The sequence analysis was done by using an automated Edman degradation system to determine the N-terminal protein sequence. An aliquot of each successive degradation was analyzed for PTH-amino acid derivatives. The resulting N-terminal amino acid sequence of the material through 15 positions showed 2 bST sequences. The sequences were present at close to an equimolar ratio. One sequence was homologous to the N-terminus of the bST protein, and the other sequence represented a fragment produced by cleavage at the same site as the thrombin cleavage site as shown in Figure 1. Thus, the exact position of the cleavage site was between amino acid 132 and 133, which is identical to the thrombin cleavage site. Therefore, the major identified metabolite of bST in plasma following sometribove administration was the same as the thrombin-clipped bST.

RESIDUE STUDIES

Bovine Somatotropin

Cattle Milk

Several milk residue studies were conducted to determine if bST concentrations are increased when animals were treated with somidobove. In the first experiment (Schams and Karg, 1988b), eight cows (4 controls and 4 treated) of different breeds were used. Treated animals were injected subcutaneously with 640 mg of somidobove every 28 days. Bovine ST milk concentrations in the controls and all treated animals were below the detection limit of the assay of 0.5 ng/ml in skim milk.

In an overdosing study (Kline et al., 1987), seventeen lactating Holstein heifers, divided in four treatment groups, were used. The four treatment groups were made up of: control (n=5), 960 mg of somidobove (n=8), 2880 mg of somidobove, and 4800 mg of somidobove. Milk samples were taken from each animal on two occasions before the injection and at 2 day intervals until 28 days after injection. The milk was assayed for bST content by RIA, with a sensitivity limit of 1.6 ng/ml bST in milk. Bovine ST concentrations in milk samples were below the sensitivity limit of the assay for all control animals and all animals treated with 960 mg of somidobove. One milk sample from a heifer treated with 2880 mg of somidobove was assayed at 2.2 ng somatotropin/ml and four samples from the animals treated with 4800 mg were assayed at somatotropin levels up to 2.75 ng/ml.

In the last study (Smith et al., 1985), six lactating dairy cows were given either no treatment (3 controls) or a subcutaneous injection containing 960 mg of somidobove in the sustained-release formulation. Milk samples were collected pre-treatment and at daily intervals for 14 days following treatment. The milk was assayed for total somatotropin content by RIA with a test sensitivity of 0.9 ng/ml. No somatotropin was detected above the sensitivity limit of the method in any milk sample from the treated cows.

In these residue studies, levels of bST in the milk of cows treated with up to 960 mg somidobove every 28 days did not result in detectable residues of somatotropin as measured by the RIA with a sensitivity of 0.9-1.6 ng/ml. These studies demonstrate that the use of bST will not lead to any detectable residues in milk above 0.9-1.6 ng/ml.

Cattle Tissues

Five lactating dairy cows were administered 500 mg of sometribove every 14 days. While on treatment, the muscle and liver of the cows were biopsied at each of the following times: after the first injection, 7 days after the first injection, after the second injection (day 14), 7 days after the second injection (day 21), and after the third injection (day 28). The samples were analyzed using validated RIA procedures. The results are summarized in Table 1. (Hammond et al., 1990).

Table 1. Concentration of bST (ppb) in Biopsied Tissues of Dairy Cattle Injected with 500 mg of Sometribove

Withdrawal	Muscle		Liver	
Time (days)	Control	Treated	Control	Treated
0	2.6 ± 2.1[a]	2.8 ± 1.3	13 ± 2.5	16 ± 3.8
7	2.1 ± 1.9	3.1 ± 1.7	11 ± 2.1	24 ± 9.5
14	2.9 ± 1.8	4.0 ± 2.2	12 ± 2.6	18 ± 7.4
21	3.7 ± 2.7	4.2 ± 2.2	11 ± 3.6	25 ± 5.6
28	2.1 ± 1.7	3.7 ± 0.7	9 ± 3.0	16 ± 6.8

[a]Values are means ± SD.

Based on the data, sometribove treatment of cows leads, at most, to a 2-fold increase in bST concentrations in muscle and liver.

INSULIN-LIKE GROWTH FACTOR-I

Cattle Milk

Monsanto conducted several studies to determine the average baseline concentration of IGF-I in untreated cow's milk. White et al. (1989a) estimated the range of IGF-I concentration typically found in bulk tank milk from dairy cows.

A survey of of 100 raw bulk tank milk samples from a commercial processing plant was conducted to provide additional data on the naturally-occurring range of IGF-I concentrations in milk. The mean IGF-I concentration in these samples was 4.32 ng/ml with a range of 1.27-8.10 ng/ml.

Collier et al. (1988) estimated the range of IGF-I concentrations found in milk from Missouri dairy cows. Milk samples from 408 untreated cows from five Missouri dairy herds were assayed for IGF-I concentrations by RIA, which had a sensitivity of 0.05 ng/ml. The highest mean concentration of IGF-I in milk was detected in early lactation (days 6-15, 6.2 ng/ml) after which milk concentrations declined. Lowest values were detected at mid-lactation (days 150-210, 1.85 ng/ml) after which they increased slightly (210+ days, 2.22 ng/ml). Older animals had significantly higher mean milk IGF-I concentrations (2.83 ng/ml) than first lactation animals (2.15 ng/ml). However, stage of lactation effects were detected in both parities and the effect of parity was apparent at all stages of lactation.

Considerable variation in milk IGF-I concentrations was related to the farm that the milk was collected from (range of farm means, 0.74-4.21 ng/ml). This significance was not related to an unequal representation of parities, stage of lactation or level of milk production from each of the farms.

The survey studies show that the levels of IGF-I in milk of untreated cows is quite variable ranging from 0.7 to 8.1 ng/ml, depending on parity and stage of lactation of the cow.

Schams and Karg (1988b, 1988c) investigated the increase in IGF-I concentrations in the milk of cows treated with somidobove. In the first experiment, eight cows (4 controls and 4 treated) of different breeds were used. The treated cows were injected subcutaneously with 640 mg of somidobove every 28 days. Milk was collected in the morning before the 3rd injection and further on days 1, 3, 6, 8, 10, 13, 15, 17, 20, 22, 24, 27 and after the 4th injection of bST on days 1, 3, 6, 8, 10 and 13.

After somidobove injection, mean IGF-I levels in the treated animals are always higher than those found in the controls. The average IGF-I milk concentration found in the control animals was 28.4 ng/ml, and the average IGF-I milk concentration in the 640 mg somidobove-treated animals was 35.5 ng/ml. Therefore, in this study an increase of approximately 25% of the mean was found in the somidobove-treated animals. It should be noted that concentrations of IGF-I in skim milk from treated cows are less than 5% of those measured in the blood plasma (1000 ng/ml).

In a study conducted for Elanco (Davis et al., 1989), thirty-six cows (24 Friesian, 12 Jersey), weighing approximately 420 kg, that had completed at least one full lactation, were used. Somidobove was given in a single subcutaneous injection at three different doses to the three different groups (12 cows/group): zero (vehicle), 320 mg and 640 mg. A composite milk sample was taken for IGF-I determination at 3, 10, 17 and 24 days after treatment at consecutive p.m. and a.m. milkings.

The concentration of IGF-I in milk was higher by day 3 in cows treated with 320 and 640 mg of somidobove relative to the control cows. The values at day 10 and thereafter were not significantly different between treatment groups. In the day 3 milk samples, the IGF-I concentrations ranged from 8-14 ng/ml in control cows, 6-32 ng/ml in the 320 mg dose group, and 9-19 ng/ml in the 640 mg dose group. One cow in the 640 mg dose group showed consistently high values for milk IGF-I content. Values on days 3, 10, 17 and 24 were 27, 58, 26 and 16 ng/ml, respectively. After somidobove treatment in this study, the levels of IGF-I in the milk increased less than 50% relative to the milk IGF-I content in the control cows.

Torkelson et al. (1988) compared concentrations of IGF-I in untreated cows to IGF-I concentrations in sometribove-treated cows. To assess the impact of bST treatment on milk IGF-I, samples were collected from 9 control cows and 9 cows treated with 500 mg of sometribove every 14 days in a prolonged-release formulation. Milk samples were collected 7 days after each of the 3 consecutive treatments. After each of the 3 doses, mean milk IGF-I in controls was 3.22, 2.62 and 3.78 ng/ml and in treated cows was 3.80, 5.39 and 4.98 ng/ml, respectively. Differences between treated and control groups was significant after the second and third doses. However, concentrations of IGF-I in milk from bST-treated animals were within the range of values detected in milk from untreated cows.

White et al. (1989b) conducted a study to provide additional data relative to the effect of exogenous administration of oil-formulated sometribove on milk concentrations of IGF-I. Eighteen lactating Holstein cows were randomly divided into two groups of nine each and administered subcutaneous injections of 500 mg of sometribove in a prolonged-release formulation or a sham injection at a 14-day interval.

Milk IGF-I concentrations also significantly increased in the sometribove treated animals although the increases were numerically small and occurred only in injection cycles two and three of treatment. The overall range of concentration for both treatment groups were similar with the control group having a range of 2.16-8.15 ng/ml and the sometribove treatment group having a range of 1.56-8.83 ng/ml. These results are summarized in Table 2.

Table 2. Least-squares means for ln and actual milk IGF-I concentrations and the numerical range of IGF-I levels (ng/ml)

Sample	Treatment	Ln Conc.*	± SEM	Mean**	Range
Pretreatment	Control	1.62	± 0.11	5.05	3.01 - 9.04
	500 mg rbGH	1.37	± 0.11	3.95	0.84 - 7.53
Day 7	Control	1.15	± 0.08	3.17	2.85 - 4.29
	500 mg rbGH	1.25	± 0.07	3.50	1.56 - 7.05
Day 21	Control	1.21	± 0.14	3.34	2.04 - 5.79
	500 mg rbGH	1.67†	± 0.14	5.33†	2.67 - 8.83
Day 35	Control	1.21	± 0.11	3.35	2.16 - 8.15
	500 mg rbGH	1.54†	± 0.11	4.68†	3.23 - 7.38

*Least-squares means ± SEM of least-squares means; **Mean = Antilog of log concentration; †These means are significantly different from the control values ($P < 0.05$).

Miller et al. (1989a) assessed the potential carryover of IGF-I in processed milk. IGF-I concentrations were measured in raw and pasteurized milk and in milk treated using conditions similar to those used in the preparation of infant formula (autoclaving).

Daily milk samples were obtained before and after pasteurization from a local commercial processing plant. The milk was pasteurized using a standard procedure. Conditions used to process milk for infant formula, i.e. heating in a retort at 250°F for 15 minutes, can be simulated in the laboratory by autoclaving milk at similar temperatures for comparable times. Raw (unpasteurized) and pasteurized milk samples were subjected to conditions simulating retorting and then assayed for IGF-I content. These results were then compared to measured IGF-I in actual Similac® infant formula milk.

The raw milk and pasteurized milk samples contained measurable levels of IGF-I of 5.6 and 8.2 ng/ml, respectively. The infant formula contained only trace amounts of IGF-I of 0.7 ng/ml. These results suggest that IGF-I is not destroyed by the pasteurization process but the heating of milk for the preparation of infant formula denatures IGF-I.

When the raw or pasteurized milk samples were heat-treated using a process similar to that of infant formula, the amount of IGF-I remaining in the milk was below detection and at least one-fifth of the preheat-treatment concentrations.

American Cyanamid conducted an extensive study of the effect of stage of lactation, diet composition and daily injections of somagrebove to Holstein cows on concentrations of IGF-I in milk (Schingoethe and Cleale, 1989). Twenty multiparous cows were assigned to one of four treatments with each treatment group containing 5 cows each. The four treatments consisted of two control groups, one fed a normal diet and the other fed a high energy and protein diet with both groups receiving excipient only, and the other two treatment groups, one fed a normal diet and the other fed a high energy and protein diet with both receiving 10.3 mg somagrebove daily. The treatments began 28-35 days postpartum and continued for 16 weeks.

Milk samples were collected every Monday p.m. and Tuesday a.m. of the treatment period and assayed for IGF-I content by RIA. Concentrations of immunoreactive IGF-I were not statistically different ($P > 0.89$) in milk of somagrebove-treated cows collected from consecutive p.m. and a.m. milkings. The mean IGF-I concentration throughout the study in the control animals was 9.67 ng/ml and in the somagrebove-treated animals was 9.06 ng/ml. Concentrations of IGF-I were significantly higher ($P < 0.05$) in the milk from the cows that consumed the high energy and protein diet than those that received the normal diet. Therefore, this study demonstrates that there is no increase in IGF-I concentration in the milk of cows treated with up to 10.3 mg of somagrebove when tested for a 16 week period.

Elanco also conducted a study to determine the concentration of IGF-I in the raw milk of control cows and the raw, pasteurized and heat-treated milk of cows receiving sustained release somidobove. In addition, the concentration of IGF-I was determined in commercially available pasteurized milk and infant formulae (Coleman et al., 1990).

Six multiparous and six primiparous Holstein cows were used in the study. Primiparous cows ranged from two to four years of age and weighed from 553 to 607 kg. Multiparous cows ranged in age from four to eight years and weighed from 649 to 689 kg. Animals were randomly assigned to treatment or control groups based on parity. The treatment group (three primiparous and three multiparous cows) received 640 mg somidobove in a sustained release vehicle in two doses, 28 days apart.

The milk from each cow was collected before injection and on days 3, 10, 17 and 24 after each injection. Raw milk samples were refrigerated pending analysis. The concentrations of IGF-I in the milk samples were determined using an RIA procedure.

In addition to the raw milk samples, milk from supplemented cows collected on days 3 and 10 of the second treatment period was pasteurized and heat-treated, and analyzed for IGF-I using the RIA method. The method had a sensitivity limit of 1 ng/ml. Pasteurized milk was heated to $63 \pm 2^{\circ}C$ for 30 minutes *as per* the Pasteurized Milk Ordinance. Heat-treated milk was autoclaved at $121 \pm 2^{\circ}C$, 19 ± 2 psi for five minutes. Heat-treated samples were analyzed at 1, 6 and 24 hours after heat treatment to demonstrate that IGF-I was permanently denatured by the treatment and did not renature after cooling to ambient temperature.

IGF-I concentrations in the milk of treated and control cows for each specified day through two injection periods are shown in Table 3.

Table 3. Concentration of IGF-I (ng/ml) in the Milk of Control and Somidobove-treated Cows for Each Specified Day Through Two Injection Periods

Injection Period	Day Post-injection	IGF-I [mean ± SD]	
		Control	Somidobove
Pretreatment	- -	19.8 ± 4.0	22.2 ± 7.6
1	3	18.0 ± 3.1	22.2 ± 4.7
1	10	21.6 ± 3.4	26.7 ± 6.3
1	17	22.7 ± 4.8	22.8 ± 5.8
1	24	21.3 ± 4.9	18.4 ± 3.6
2	3	21.0 ± 2.8	23.8 ± 4.8
2	10	26.3 ± 6.6	30.8 ± 8.6
2	17	25.3 ± 6.8	23.4 ± 4.5
2	24	24.4 ± 5.8	23.0 ± 3.7

It should be noted that IGF-I concentrations in raw milk samples are similar for cows of different parities and different treatment-parity combinations. Table 4 demonstrates the effect of pasteurization and heat treatment on the IGF-I levels in the milk of somidobove-treated cattle. Table 5 contains information on the concentration of IGF-I in 3 brands of commercially available pasteurized milk and 3 brands of infant formulae.

Table 4. IGF-I Concentrations (ng/ml) in the Milk of Somidobove-treated Cattle Following Pasteurization and Heat Treatment

Milk Treatment	Hours Post-treatment	IGF-I [mean ± SD]
None	0	24.1 ± 4.3
Pasteurized	1	23.9 ± 4.1
	6	29.5 ± 5.1
	24	27.5 ± 4.0
Heat-treated	1	14.3 ± 2.6
	6	14.2 ± 1.9
	24	12.9 ± 2.4

The sponsor concludes that pasteurization has no effect on the concentration of IGF-I in milk. Autoclaved milk, simulating processing for infant formulae, had significantly reduced (35 - 48%) levels of IGF-I compared to raw milk.

Table 5. Concentration of IGF-I (ng/ml) in Commercially Available Pasteurized Milk and Infant Formulae

	IGF-I [mean ± SD]
3 Brands of Milk	
A	25.5 ± 6.5
B	25.0 ± 4.4
C	23.6 ± 4.6
Brand of Formula	
1	13.6 ± 3.4
+ 50 ng IGF-I/ml	83.2 ± 9.7
2	16.3 ± 1.6
+ 50 ng IGF-I/ml	78.2 ± 9.3
3	7.3 ± 2.2
+ 50 ng IGF-I/ml	69.7 ± 5.3

Monsanto also conducted a milk residue study to determine if an increase in IGF-II concentrations existed in sometribove-treated cows. Sixty-four lactating Holstein cows (21 primiparous, 43 multiparous) were used in the study and the animals either received 500 mg sometribove in an oil-based prolonged release formulation or excipient via intramuscular or subcutaneous injection at 14 day intervals. Treatments were administered from 60 ± 3 days postpartum until a minimum of

74 days prior to expected calving or until a cow's average daily milk production for an injection cycle dropped below 5 kg/day (when dry-off occurred). Milking was done twice daily at 0600 and 1800 hours. Composite milk samples from each cow were collected on day -7 of the pretreatment period and on day 7 of injection cycles 1-10.

Milk concentration of IGF-I was increased across the 10 injection cycles. The average increase in milk IGF-I concentration was 2.2 ng/ml and there was no parity by treatment interaction. There was no increase in milk IGF-II concentrations in any of the sampling periods (Table 6). (Miller et al., 1989b)

Table 6. The effect of 500 mg of sometribove administered intramuscularly (IM) or subcutaneously (SC) on milk concentrations of IGF-I and IGF-II (*least squares means ± SEM).

Sampling Period	Primiparous Cows		Multiparous Cows	
	Milk IGF-I Concentration* (ng/ml)			
Overall Cycle 1-10				
Control	3.5	(± 0.67)	3.9	(± 0.39)
IM	5.9†	(± 0.59)	5.9†	(± 0.37)
SC	6.1†	(± 0.60)	5.6†	(± 0.39)
	Milk IGF-II Concentration* (ng/ml)			
Overall Cycle 1-10				
Control	106.6	(± 9.11)	97.8	(± 6.21)
IM	116.3	(± 8.47)	107.2	(± 5.99)
SC	116.4	(± 8.36)	94.5	(± 5.95)

†These means are significantly different from the control values (*P* < 0.05, protected t-test).

In summary, the biweekly injection of 500 mg of sometribove in lactating cattle increased milk IGF-I concentrations. However, there was no increase in milk IGF-II concentrations in milk from bST-treated animals.

<u>Cattle Tissues</u>

Five lactating dairy cows were administered 500 mg of sometribove every 14 days. While on treatment, the muscle and liver of the cows were biopsied at each of the following times: after the first injection, 7 days after the first injection, after the second injection (day 14), 7 days after the second injection (day 21), and after the third injection (day 28). The samples were analyzed using validated RIA procedures. The results of this study are summarized in Table 7. (Hammond et al., 1990).

Table 7. Concentration of IGF-I (ppb) in Biopsied Tissues of Dairy Cattle Injected with 500 mg of Sometribove

Withdrawal	Muscle		Liver	
Time (days)	Control	Treated	Control	Treated
0	80 ± 16[a]	91 ± 26	77 ± 6.2	72 ± 9.0
7	272 ± 160[b]	312 ± 130	72 ± 9.1	162 ± 36
14	252 ± 141	152 ± 62	72 ± 15	112 ± 11
21	68 ± 20	126 ± 58	70 ± 8.3	142 ± 52
28	215 ± 173	135 ± 19	70 ± 14	92 ± 15

[a]Values are means ± SD
[b]Elevated IGF-I levels are associated with wound healing as biopsies at these intervals were collected from the same anatomical locations (Jennische et al., 1987).

Human Milk

Human milk concentrations of IGF-I were measured during the first 9 days postpartum (Baxter et al., 1984). The mean IGF-I concentration at 1-day postpartum was 17.6 ng/ml, at 2-days postpartum was 12.8 ng/ml and at 3-days postpartum was 6.8 ng/ml. After 3-days postpartum, the IGF-I concentration stabilized over the following week at 7-8 ng/ml. In a subsequent article (Corps et al., 1988), IGF-I concentrations in human milk were measured and ranged between 13 and 40 ng/ml at 6-8 weeks postpartum with a mean of 19 ng/ml. It was determined that IGF-I concentrations in human milk were 2- to 3-fold higher at 6- to 8-weeks postpartum than that 3-7 days postpartum.

METHODS OF ANALYSIS FOR RESIDUES IN TISSUES

The analytical methods used to determine the amount of bST and IGF-I in the plasma, milk and tissue of the cow were exclusively immunoassay procedures, primarily RIA (Collier et al., 1991; Malven et al., 1987; Torkelson et al., 1987). Each sponsor developed their own immunoassay; none could distinguish between the natural bST and their recombinant bST product. All procedures were validated and extensively evaluated. The 2-3 fold difference seen in the concentrations of bST and IGF-I between companies reflect differences in the antisera and differences in the purity of the reference standard used (Grings et al., 1988). When rbST standard is used, values are approximately 3.3 times lower than values ontained with NIH standards.

APPRAISAL

There are 4 different recombinantly derived bST (rbST) products being evaluated by the Committee. They either slightly differed in the N-terminal portion of the protein from pituitary bST or are identical in amino acid sequence. Treatment of lactating dairy cows with rbST causes an increase in plasma bST concentrations and milk production which is physiologically indistinguishable from the changes induced with pituitary-derived bST. The analytical methods used to determine the concentration of bST in plasma, milk or tissues do not differentiate between rbST and endogenous bST. Thus, when concentrations of bST are given, they are total bST concentrations.

Milk residue studies demonstrate, even at exaggerated doses, that the proposed use of rbST will not lead to any detectable concentrations of bST in milk above those normally present in untreated cows (0.9-1.6 μg/L). Additionally, the major metabolite identified in the serum was the same as the bST fragment cleaved by thrombin, between amino acid 132 and 133.

In regard to tissue residue data, rbST treatment of cows leads, at most, to a 2-fold increase in bST concentrations to levels of 4.2 μg/kg in muscle and 25 μg/kg in liver.

Some studies suggest that rbST treatment may produce a slight increase in the average milk IGF-I (insulin-like growth factor I) concentration; however, the most definitive and comprehensive studies demonstrate that IGF-I concentrations are not altered after rbST treatment. Additionally, IGF-II concentrations in cows' milk are also not affected by rbST treatment.

Further results indicate that rbST is denatured after pasteurization, but IGF-I is not destroyed by the pasteurization process. However, the heating of milk for the preparation of infant formula reduces the amount of IGF-I by at least 50%. Additionally, human breast milk contains IGF-I concentrations which are similar to those found in control and rbST-treated cows.

IGF-I concentrations in the biopsied muscle and liver of rbST-treated cows increase at most 2-fold to 300 and 160 mg/kg, respectively. However, these elevated IGF-I concentrations in the muscle may not be related to rbST treatment but to wound healing.

The effects of rbST on the major components of milk, if any, are minor and primarily occur early in the treatment period prior to adjustments in dry matter intake by the cow. Furthermore, milk composition of treated cows is well within the normal variation observed during the course of a lactation. Thus, there appears to be no significant impact of rbST treatment on the nutritional and processing qualities of milk.

APPENDIX

Effects of bST Treatment of Cows on Milk Composition

Milk and dairy products can serve as major source of nutrients for both children and adults and are particularly high in protein, calcium, phosphorus, and several vitamins. The unique biophysical properties of milk also impact its processing into various dairy products. Thus, any production drug, feed, or management technique proposed for dairy cows would be of questionable value if it adversely altered the nutritive and processing qualities of milk.

The physiology and biochemistry of milk synthesis in dairy cows do not appear to be significantly changed due to bST. Studies evaluating the energy metabolism of dairy cows treated with rbST suggest that nutrient digestibility, maintenance requirements, and the utilization of metabolizable energy for milk production are unchanged. Rather, more nutrients are directed toward milk synthesis as opposed to tissue deposition (Bauman et al., 1985; Tyrrell et al., 1988; Kirchgessner et al., 1989; Sechen et al., 1989; McGuffey et al., 1991).

Early experiments reported in the literature (c. 1980-1985) suggested no direct effects of short-term bST treatment of dairy cows on fat, protein, lactose, calcium, and phosphorus content of milk. However, evaluation under proposed conditions for use is an important aspect of the review of production drugs. For this reason the drug sponsors were requested to submit data from repeated sampling and analysis of milk composition throughout full lactation studies of effectiveness and animal safety of rbST.

Numerous reports of experiments which evaluated the effects of rbST on milk production and general composition have been published. Some researchers have also examined in detail the chemical composition and processing qualities of milk from rbST-treated cows. This section will focus primarily on published reports in addition to abstracts which specifically address the composition of milk from rbST-treated cows.

Lipid Components. The majority of the lipid component of bovine milk is composed of triglycerides (97-98%). Remaining lipids include diglycerides, monoglycerides, free fatty acids, phospholipids, cholesterol, and other components in minute quantities. Fat content in fresh milk is the most variable of its major components and is dependent upon a number of factors such as diet, stage of lactation, season, and environment. Differences also exist among breeds of cattle. Holsteins, the predominant breed in the U.S., have the lowest milk fat content (about 3.6%), whereas Jerseys produce milk with the highest concentration (about 5.0%; Jenness, 1985).

Dietary changes are probably the easiest way to manipulate milk fat content. The main precursors of bovine milk fat are affected by diet through changes in rumen fermentation and availability of endogenous fatty acid sources. In particular, feeding rations high in readily fermentable carbohydrates (grain) and low in fiber (forage) to increase energy content of the ration may depress rumen pH. Rumen fermentation in turn is altered such that fatty acid precursors are reduced. In extreme cases, milk fat percent may be reduced as much as 60 percent. The physical form of forages in the diet also has an influence of fat percent; for example, finely ground, immature, or low fiber forages may depress rumen pH and reduce milk fat content. Some of these negative effects of highly fermentable feeds on milk fat percentages may be minimized by adding buffers to diets to increase rumen pH (Linn, 1988).

Concentrations of milk fat also vary in cows over stage of lactation. Milk fat percent of colostrum is relatively high (>5%) and then decreases until about 5 to 10 weeks postpartum (about 3.6%), at which point fat content increases until the end of lactation (approximately 45 weeks) to about 4% (Jenness, 1985). Part of this variation can be attributed to the high grain diets typically fed to cows in early lactation to maximize energy consumption during peak lactation. However, the high milk volume in early lactation also dilutes fat concentration.

Other factors influencing milk fat composition include age and seasonal changes. Fat content of milk decreases as cows become older and on average is 0.4 percentage units lower during summer months than in cooler seasons, although diet may confound seasonal effects (Jenness, 1985; Linn, 1988).

Peak daily milk yield in the dairy cow occurs at approximately 4 to 8 weeks postpartum and then gradually decreases. Voluntary feed intake follows a similar pattern, but maximum intake occurs between 10 and 14 weeks postpartum. Thus, cows are typically in negative energy balance in the first two months of lactation and mobilize considerable amounts of adipose tissue to supply the tremendous amounts of energy needed to sustain high levels of milk production during early lactation. Increased circulating concentrations of nonesterified fatty acids (NEFA) due to mobilization of adipose tissue can increase milk fat percentages. Adipose tissue stores are typically replenished in late lactation as daily milk yields diminish over time (NRC, 1989).

Milk that is commercially available does not reflect the natural variation in fat content among cows since standardization to various fat levels is a regular part of the commercial processing of milk.

Effects of bST on milk fat percent are dependent upon the energy balance of the treated animal. An increase in milk yield typically occurs within 5 days after initiation of treatment. When milk production response causes the animal to be in negative energy balance, milk fat percent is usually increased due to mobilization of adipose tissue (Bauman et al., 1988) and increased plasma concentrations of NEFA (Eppard et al., 1985a; Peel and Bauman, 1987; Bauman et al., 1988; Lough et al., 1988; Van den Berg, 1989). In contrast, when bST-treated cows were consuming sufficient quantities of nutrients to meet the energy needs for additional milk synthesis, body lipid mobilization did not increase, but lipid synthesis was instead reduced (Sechen et al., 1989). In this scenario, blood levels of NEFA were unchanged, and milk fat content was also unaffected (Eppard et al., 1985a; Peel and Bauman, 1987; Sechen et al., 1989; Van den Berg, 1989).

Long-term administration of rbST to dairy cows usually results in increased voluntary dry matter intake after approximately 5 to 10 weeks of treatment to support increased milk synthesis (Bauman et al., 1985; 1989; Elvinger et al., 1988; Soderholm et al., 1988). Depending on the stage of lactation when treatment is initiated and dose of rbST administered, cows will typically be in negative, or at least reduced, energy balance in the first few weeks of treatment until the adjustment in intake (Bauman et al., 1985; 1989; Elvinger et al., 1988; Baer et al., 1989), and milk fat percent may be increased during this period (Baer et al., 1989). Most studies indicate that milk fat percentages averaged over the entire rbST treatment period are no different than controls (Bauman et al., 1985; 1989; Elvinger et al., 1988; Soderholm et al., 1988; Baer et al., 1989; Van den Berg, 1989). Lean et al. (1991) found that cows treated with relatively high doses of a daily injectable rbST product in their previous lactation tended to have lower milk fat percentages than controls in the early postpartum period (i.e., before rbST treatment resumed). This was probably due to the fact that the formerly treated cows had maintained higher dry matter intake and energy balance than controls and lower serum NEFA concentrations during the postpartum period.

In most mammalian tissues the predominant fatty acid synthesized is palmitic acid (16:0). However, enzymes in the mammary gland are modified to permit synthesis of shorter chain fatty acids. The fatty acids between 4 and 15 carbons in length as well as about 50% of C16 fatty acids are synthesized de novo within the mammary gland. The remaining C16 and all of the longer fatty acids are derived from dietary sources or body lipid stores. The net effect is that approximately 50% of milk fatty acids are between 4 and 16 carbons in length, and the remaining fatty acids are predominantly 18 carbons long. Greater than 95% of these fatty acids in bovine milk are found in triglycerides (Jenness, 1985).

Similar to fat percent, effects of rbST treatment on fatty acid composition in milk appears to depend on energy balance of the treated cow. In general, when production responses due to bST treatment result in negative energy balance, adipose tissue mobilization increases, resulting in a smaller proportion of short- to medium-chain fatty acids (less than 16 carbons in length) and more long-chain fatty acids (16 and 18 carbons) in milk fat. If energy consumption is sufficient to maintain positive energy balance, proportions of fatty acids do not change (Bitman et al., 1984; Eppard et al., 1985b; Lough et al., 1988; Van den Berg, 1989). Lynch et al. (1988a) demonstrated that shifts in fatty acid composition of milk with stage of lactation were the same in both treated and control cows (treatment beginning at 60 days postpartum). In early lactation when both groups of cows were in negative energy balance, the percentage of short-chain fatty acids in milk was lower, whereas long-chain fatty acids were higher in concentration. As cows returned to positive energy balance after 8 to 12 weeks of lactation, these changes were reversed. The changes due to stage of lactation were independent of rbST treatment. Differences in proportions of fatty acids in milk of treated cows as compared to controls are only evident early in the treatment period prior to adjustments in feed intake (Lynch et al., 1988a; Baer et al., 1989; Van den Berg, 1989). Lean et al. (1991) reported lower ratios of long-chain to short-chain fatty acids in milk during the early subsequent lactation period in cows treated with high doses of bST on a daily basis in their previous lactation compared to controls. The formerly treated cows were consuming more feed and were in higher energy balance that controls during this period and presumably mobilizing less body lipid.

The normal cholesterol content of milk lipid is approximately 0.2 to 0.4 percent (Jenness, 1985). Bitman et al. (1984) observed a significant decrease in milk cholesterol content in cows treated with rbST for 14 days and in negative energy balance (0.34 vs. 0.27% of milk lipid). However, over a longer period of treatment (days 60 through 305 of lactation), Lynch et al. (1989a) found that cholesterol content of milk fat was similar between control and rbST-treated cows, 33.1 and 34.6 mg per cup of whole milk, respectively, or approximately one-ninth of the recommended daily intake of cholesterol (300 mg/day). Once again, stage of lactation had the greatest effect on milk cholesterol content; levels increased in both control and treated cows as lactation progressed.

To summarize, treatment of cows with rbST does not create new and unusual fatty acids in milk, nor does it affect cholesterol content. During long-term treatment with rbST, changes in proportions of fatty acids are minor and return to control levels once dry matter intake adjusts and nutrient requirements to support increased milk yields are met. Stage of lactation has a much greater effect on fatty acid and cholesterol content in milk than rbST treatment.

Total Protein (Nitrogen) Fraction. Total protein in milk includes various caseins, whey proteins (e.g., lactoglobulin, lactalbumin, albumin, immunoglobulins) and nonprotein nitrogen (e.g., peptides, amino acids, urea, ammonia). Total protein percent of fresh milk (i.e., nitrogen times 6.38) often shows considerable variation, although not to as great an extent as fat. Among breeds, Holsteins average 3.2% protein, whereas milk from Jerseys is typically around 3.8%. Total protein content in bovine colostrum is high (about 16%), primarily due to increased immunoglobulin concentrations. This quickly reduces to approximately 3.5% within 5 days postpartum. Milk protein content reduces to approximately 3.0% at 5 to 10 weeks postpartum, and then increases to 4.0% towards the end of lactation, thus corresponding inversely to milk yield (Jenness, 1985).

Insufficient amounts of dietary protein will reduce milk protein concentration, although the source protein in the diet may also have an effect. Similar to fat percent, protein in milk tends to decrease as cows age. High temperatures also have a negative effect on milk protein content (Jenness, 1985; Linn, 1988).

The percent total protein in milk of cows treated with bST appears to be dependent primarily upon resultant nitrogen balance. A number of studies have demonstrated that if treatment results in a negative or significantly reduced nitrogen balance, protein content of milk is reduced, indicative of a limited supply of amino acids (Eppard et al., 1985a; Peel and Bauman, 1987; Bauman et al., 1988; Baer et al., 1989; Van den Berg, 1989). In contrast, if positive nitrogen balance is maintained, the protein content of milk usually does not change (see Eppard et al., 1985a; Peel and Bauman, 1987; Lough et al., 1988; Sechen et al., 1989; Van den Berg, 1989). In long-term treatment with daily injectable rbST products (5 to 40 mg/day), feed intake adjusts to meet nutrient requirements for extra milk production, and milk protein percent over the lactation is not significantly altered from controls (Bauman et al., 1985; Elvinger et al., 1988; Leonard et al., 1988; Soderholm et al., 1988; Baer et al., 1989). An exception was the study by Kindstedt et al. (1991) in which Jersey cows treated with 500 mg bST/14 days starting 8 weeks postpartum until the end of lactation had significantly lower total milk protein than controls (3.92 vs. 4.12%) averaged over the entire treatment period despite being higher in average protein balance during the same period. Nevertheless, stage of lactation had a greater effect on milk protein percent that bST treatment (Elvinger et al., 1988; Leonard et al., 1988; Kindstedt et al., 1991).

Milk protein percent (and milk fat content to a lesser extent) in cows treated with sustained release rbST products shows a cyclic pattern; the percent tends to be higher in the latter phase of the injection cycle, i.e., the last few days of 14-day cycles and week 4 with 28-day sustained release products (Bauman et al., 1989; Van den Berg, 1989). Milk yield also had a cyclic pattern with these sustained release products, with peak yield occurring during the first half of each cycle. Since milk protein percent during the "valleys" of cycles in rbST-treated cows did not fall below control levels the changes did not appear to be related to nitrogen balance. Rather, different half-lives for enzymatic processes related to milk synthesis may vary (Bauman et al., 1989). For example, if enzymatic changes related to lactose production (and therefore milk volume, see below) had shorter half-lives as compared to those related to fat and protein synthesis, expected changes in milk volume would result in the observed patterns. Indeed, milk lactose concentration was relatively constant during injection intervals (Bauman et al., 1989).

Because of the cycling of total protein percent in milk of cows treated with sustained release rbST products, interpretation of the effect on protein content may be influenced by the days in which milk samples are collected. Bauman et al. (1989), who sampled milk on days 5 and 12 of each 14-day cycle, reported increased content of total protein in milk (3.34 vs. 3.25%) when cows were treated with 500 mg rbST/cycle. Kindstedt et al. (1991) found total milk protein to be lower in Jersey cows injected every 14 days with 500 mg rbST. Milk was sampled on day 8 of the cycle, when milk protein was expected to be lowest in treated cows. Nevertheless, Ozimak et al. (1989) observed the opposite effect despite a similar sampling schedule as Kindstedt et al. (1991); total protein content was higher in milk of treated cows than in milk of controls (350 mg rbST/14 days; 3.52 vs. 3.27%) with sampling on day 7 of the 14-day cycle. Lenoir and Schockmel (1987) measured no differences in total protein of milk from cows treated with rbST on a biweekly basis versus controls. However, milk was sampled once per month on a calendar basis over 6 months, and therefore, was not synchronized with injection cycles. This suggests that cycling of milk protein with sustained-release products would likely have little influence on commingled milk from different farms since cows are at different stages of lactation and would be on different injection schedules.

Approximately 95% of the total nitrogen fraction in bovine milk is found in true proteins, and in general, this fraction provides the majority of the nutritional quality of milk with respect to protein. Milk proteins are generally subdivided into two classes: caseins and whey proteins.

Caseins are unique to milk and make up approximately 80% of the true protein in bovine milk (Jenness, 1985). There are several types of caseins including alpha- (several variants), beta-, gamma-, and kappa-casein which, along with fat content, determine the potential yield and quality of cheese produced from a volume of milk. For example, curd formation is triggered by specific proteolysis of kappa-casein, and adequate separation of whey from curds is dependent upon beta-casein (see review by Pearse and Mackinlay, 1989).

A number of studies examining casein content, expressed as a percent of milk, in cows treated with rbST over a full lactation demonstrated no differences from control levels (Lenoir and Schockmel, 1987; Leonard et al., 1988; Barbano et al., 1988; Baer et al., 1989; Van den Berg, 1989). Ozimek et al. (1989) found a significant increase in both true protein (3.17 vs. 2.88%) and casein content (2.63 vs. 2.38%) of cows treated every 14 days with 350 mg rbST. However, Kindstedt et al. (1991) reported lower true protein (3.74 vs. 3.95%) and casein (3.11 vs. 3.34%) in treated Jerseys (500 mg rbST/14 days). Baer et al. (1989) noted that true protein and casein percent tended to decrease in the first 2 weeks of treatment when cows were in negative nitrogen balance, but then returned to control levels as the lactation progressed. Indeed, stage of lactation and animal variability had more significant effects on casein composition of milk than rbST treatment (Van den Berg, 1989).

When expressed as a percent of true protein, there has been a trend toward lower casein content, e.g., 78.8 vs. 80.2% (Baer et al., 1989) and 83.38 vs. 84.52% (Kindstedt et al., 1991) in rbST treated vs. control cows, although not in all cases (Lynch et al., 1988a). This might be explained by an increase in total whey protein content in milk (Baer et al., 1989). Nevertheless, both Baer et al. (1989) and Kindstedt et al. (1991) estimated that the minor reductions in casein content they observed as a percent of true protein would amount to no more than a 0.1% lower theoretical yield of Cheddar cheese per weight of milk. Concentrations and proportions of the various casein fractions in milk of cows treated with rbST over a lactation were not different from controls (Lenoir and Schockmel, 1987; Leonard et al., 1988; Lynch et al., 1988a; Van den Berg, 1989).

Noncasein proteins in milk fall into the broad category of whey (or serum) proteins. Two of the principal whey proteins are specific products of the mammary gland: alpha-lactalbumin and beta-lactoglobulin. Other whey proteins include immunoglobulins, albumins, about 50 different enzymes, and many other compounds (Jenness, 1985).

Alpha-lactalbumin is part of the lactose synthetase complex, a rate-limiting enzyme in the synthesis of lactose, the major milk carbohydrate. It is secreted along with lactose into milk. Beta-lactoglobulin is the most abundant protein in bovine whey, but its biological function is unknown (Jenness, 1985).

Whey protein percentages in milk of cows treated with daily injectable (Leonard et al., 1988), 14-day sustained release (Lenoir and Schockmel, 1987; Kinstedt et al., 1991) or 28-day injectable rbST products (see review by Van den Berg, 1989) were not significantly different than controls. In contrast, whey protein percent was higher in a study using a daily injectable product (0.71 vs. 0.65%; Baer et al., 1989) and a 14-day injectable (0.54 vs. 0.49%, Ozimek et al., 1989). Although not measured, Baer et al. (1989) theorized that higher alpha-lactalbumin content in milk of treated cows may have increased the percent of whey protein and could explain the increase in total lactose, and consequently yield of milk, in rbST-treated cows. Indeed, Eppard et al. (1985) and Ozimek et al. (1989) reported increased alpha-lactalbumin content in milk of rbST-treated cows, although Lynch et al. (1988a) found no change as a percent of true protein. Relative percents of beta-lactoglobulin were unchanged (Lynch et al., 1988b) or higher (Ozimek et al., (1989) in rbST-treated cows.

Nonprotein nitrogen (NPN) content of bovine milk is approximately 6% of total milk nitrogen and includes amino acids, ammonia, and urea (Jenness, 1985). Nonprotein nitrogen percent or its percent of total nitrogen was higher (4.61 vs. 4.26%, Kindstedt et al., 1991; 0.179 vs. 0.172%, Barbano et al., 1988; 0.40 vs. 0.35%, Ozimek et al., 1989) or not different (Baer et al., 1989; Lenoir and Schockmel, 1987) in rbST-treated cows as opposed to controls.

Overall, results to date concerning the protein composition of milk have shown only slight, if any, alterations due to rbST treatment of cows. The type of rbST product and influence due to cycling (i.e., daily injectable vs. sustained release) and milk sampling schedule may influence interpretations. Some studies indicate a trend toward slightly increased whey proteins and NPN and decreased milk casein in rbST-treated cows. A question which remains is whether such effects are typical for cows which naturally produce more milk. Most studies over full lactations report considerably more variation due to stage of lactation than rbST treatment. The differences in milk protein composition have been small, and it appears that they would have virtually no impact on nutritional quality of milk and only minor, if any, effects on processing characteristics.

Lactose. The principle carbohydrate in the milk of most species is lactose, a disaccharide composed of glucose and galactose. Bovine milk contains approximately 4.6% lactose, and although it does vary slightly with breed of cow, stage of lactation, and climate, it is generally very constant due to its role in maintenance of milk osmolality. Overall, bST treatment has not altered lactose content in milk in short-term studies (Eppard et al., 1985; Tyrrell et al., 1988) and in studies carried out over full lactations (Bauman et al., 1985; Barbano et al., 1988). Baer et al. (1989), observed a higher concentration of lactose in milk of cows treated over a lactation (4.80 vs. 4.71%), but the minute difference is of questionable biological significance.

Minerals. While calcium and phosphorus are generally considered the most important minerals in milk, over 30 minerals have been detected. The total ash content of bovine milk averages about 0.75% (Jenness, 1985), and this was not changed in milk from cows treated with rbST over an entire lactation (Bauman et al., 1989).

Bovine milk contains approximately 1.2 g calcium and 1 g phosphorus per kg (NRC, 1989). Calcium and phosphorus content of milk of bST-treated cows are within normal ranges and show no consistent changes due to treatment (Eppard et al., 1985b; Lenoir and Schockmel, 1987; Bauman et al., 1989; Pikus et al. 1989; Van den Berg, 1989). This has similarly been demonstrated with concentrations of sodium, potassium, iron, magnesium, copper, manganese, and zinc in milk of cows treated with bST (Eppard et al., 1985b; Pikus et al., 1989; Van den Berg, 1989).

Vitamins. Milk is an important source of thiamine (vitamin B-1), riboflavin (vitamin B-2), pyridoxine (vitamin B-6), pantothenic acid, biotin, vitamin B-12, and choline. It also provides moderate amounts of niacin, folic acid, vitamins C, D, and E, and is very low in vitamin K. The bovine mammary gland cannot synthesize vitamins, so it is dependent upon its blood supply for vitamins secreted into milk. Vitamins A, D, E, and K are fat-soluble and are associated with the fat component of milk.

The B-vitamins and vitamin C are water soluble and therefore associated with the skim fraction of milk (Jenness, 1985).

Hartnell et al. (1987) measured the content of several vitamins in milk of 42 cows treated with either a placebo or sustained release rbST (500 mg/14 d). Morning milk samples collected on several days within an injection cycle were pooled per treatment group from cows at about 30 weeks postpartum and on treatment 18 to 24 weeks. Content of the following vitamins was not different in milk of rbST-treated cows as compared to controls: vitamin A, thiamine, riboflavin, pyridoxine, vitamin B-12, choline, and pantothenic acid. Biotin levels were significantly increased in milk of treated cows (0.0017 vs. 0.0019 mg/100 g), however, the small change was of questionable biological significance. Brown (1988) also determined that concentrations of vitamin A in milk of cows which were treated with rbST for a second consecutive lactation were not different than in controls.

Processing qualities and acceptability of dairy products. Van den Berg (1989) reviewed a number of U.S. and European studies evaluating the yield and quality of cheese produced from milk of rbST-treated cows. It was concluded that the manufacturing properties of milk plus yield and quality of cheeses were not affected by rbST treatment of cows.

Azzara et al. (1987), Baer et al. (1989), Lenoir and Schockmel (1987), Lynch et al. (1988b, 1989a, 1989b), and Marshall and Cartledge (1988) evaluated a number of characteristics important in the processing and stability of milk, including protease and lipase activity, starter culture growth, pH, freezing point, coagulation times, thermal properties of fat, and susceptibility to rancid flavor. No differences were detected between milk of controls and rbST-treated cows over treatment periods ranging from 6 months to a full lactation.

Taste panel evaluation of milk and cheese from rbST-treated cows has demonstrated no significant differences in taste, odor, texture, and acceptability compared to products from nontreated animals (Baer et al., 1989; Lynch et al., 1989b, Van den Berg, 1989).

Summary. The physiology and biochemistry of milk synthesis in dairy cows is not significantly altered by rbST treatment. To date, the effects of rbST on the major components of milk, if any, are minor and primarily occur early in the treatment period prior to adjustments in dry matter intake by the cow. Furthermore, milk composition of treated cows is well within the normal variation observed during the course of a lactation. Thus, there appears to be no significant impact of rbST treatment on nutritional and processing qualities of milk.

REFERENCES

Azzara, C.D., Dimick, P.S., and Chalupa, W. 1987. Milk lipoprotein lipase activity during long-term administration of recombinant bovine somatotropin. J. Dairy Sci., **70**, 1937-1940.

Baer, R.J., Tieszen, K.M., Schingoethe, D.J., Casper, D.P., Eisenbeisz, W.A., Shaver, R.D., and Cleale, R.M. 1989. Composition and flavor of milk produced by cows injected with recombinant bovine somatotropin. J. Dairy Sci., **72**, 1424-1434.

Barbano, D.M., Lynch, J.M., Bauman, D.E., and Hartnell, G.F. 1988. Influence of sometribove (recombinant methionyl bovine somatotropin) on general milk composition. J. Dairy Sci., **71**(Suppl. 1), 101.

Bauman, D.E., Eppard, P.J., DeGeeter, M.J., and Lanza, G.M. 1985. Responses of high-producing dairy cows to long-term treatment with pituitary somatotropin and recombinant somatotropin. J. Dairy Sci., **68**, 1352-1362.

Bauman, D.E., Hard, D.L., Crooker, B.A., Partridge, M.S., Garrick, K., Sandles, L.D., Erb, H.N., Franson, S.E., Hartnell, G.F., and Hintz, R.L. 1989. Long-term evaluation of a prolonged-release formulation of N-methionyl bovine somatotropin in lactating dairy cows. J. Dairy Sci., **72**, 642-651.

Bauman, D.E., Peel, C.J., Steinhour, W.D., Reynolds, P.J., Tyrrell, H.F., Brown, A.C.G., and Haaland, G.L. 1988. Effect of bovine somatotropin on metabolism of lactating dairy cows: influence on rates of irreversible loss and oxidation of glucose and nonesterified fatty acids. J. Nutr., **118**, 1031-1040.

Birmingham, B.K., White, T.C., Lanza, G.M., Miller, M.A., Torkelson, A.R., and Hale, M.D. 1988. Pharmacokinetics of sometribove (methionyl rbST) and a naturally occurring growth hormone variant in lactating dairy cows. Abstract:J. Dairy Sci., **71**, 227.

Bitman, J., Wood, D.L., Tyrrell, H.F., Bauman, D.E., Peel, C.J., Brown, A.C.G., and Reynolds, P.J. 1984. Blood and milk lipid responses induced by growth hormone administration in lactating cows. J. Dairy Sci., **67**, 2873-2880.

Brown, A.C.G. 1988. Vitamin A content of milk from animals receiving somidobove. Unpublished report T4UUK 8504/8505 dated September 14 -October 5, 1988, Lilly Research Laboratories, Greenfield, IN.

Collier, R.J., Miller, M.A., Hildebrandt, J.R., Torkelson, A.R., White, T.C., Madsen, K.S., Vicini, J.L., Eppard, P.L., and Lanza, G.M. 1991. Factors affecting Insulin-Like Growth Factor-I concentration in bovine milk, J. Dairy Sci., **74**, 2905-2911.

Collier, R.J., Torkelson, A.R., Lanza, G.M., Vicini, J.L., White, T.C., Hildebrandt, J.R., Rogan, G.J., Madsen, K.S., Eppard, P.L., Birmingham, B.K., and Malinski, T. 1988. Survey of insulin-like growth factor-I (IGF-I) concentrations in individual milk samples from five Missouri dairy herds, Unpublished report MSL 8531 dated January 6, 1988, Monsanto Agricultural Co., St. Louis, MO.

Coleman, M.R., Ghrist, B.F.D., Mowrey, D.H., McGuffey, R.K., and Kube, J.C. 1990. Determination of Insulin-like Growth Factor (IGF-I) Concentrations in Raw Milk from Non-Supplemented Animals and in Raw, Pasteurized and Heat-Treated Milk from Animals Supplemented with Somidobove, Unpublished Study T4U709001, Elanco Animal Health, Greenfield, IN.

Corps, A.N., Brown, K.D., Rees, L.H., Carr, J., and Prosser, C.G. 1988. The insulin-like growth factor 1 content in human milk increases between early and full lactation. J. Clin. Endocrinol. Metab., **67**, 25-29.

Davis, S.R., Gluckman, P.D., and Bryant, A.M. 1989. Effects of somidobove treatment of dairy cows on plasma and milk concentrations of insulin-like growth factor-I. Unpublished Elanco report, Ruakura Agricultural Centre, Hamilton, New Zealand.

Elvinger, F., Head, H.H., Wilcox, C.J., Natzke, R.P., and Eggert, R.G. 1988. Effects of administration of bovine somatotropin on milk yield and composition. J. Dairy Sci., **71**, 1515-1525.

Eppard, P.J., Bauman, D.E., and McCutcheon, S.N. 1985a. Effect of dose of bovine growth hormone on lactation of dairy cows. J. Dairy Sci., **68**, 1109-1115.

Eppard, P.J., Bauman, D.E., Bitman, J., Wood, D.L., Akers, R.M., and House, W.A. 1985b. Effect of dose of bovine growth hormone on milk composition: a-lactalbumin, fatty acids, and mineral elements. J. Dairy Sci., **68**, 3047-3054.

Grings, E.E., Scarborough, R., Schally, A.V. and Reeves, J.J. 1988. Response to a growth hormone-releasing hormone analog in heifers treated with recombinant growth hormone. Domestic Animal Endocrinology **5**(1), 47-53.

Hammond, B.G., Collier, R.J., Miller, M.A., McGrath, M., Hartzell, D.L., Kotts, C. and Vandaele, W. 1990. Food safety and pharmacokinetic studies which support a zero meat and milk withdrawal time for use of sometribove in dairy cows. Ann. Rech. Vet., **21** (Suppl. 1), 107s-120s.

Hartnell, G.F. 1987. Evaluation of vitamins in milk produced from cows treated with placebo and CP115099 in a prolonged release system. Unpublished report MSL 7031 dated May 29, 1987, Monsanto Agricultural Co., St. Louis, MO.

Jenness, R. 1985. Biochemical and nutritional aspects of milk and colostrum. In, Lactation. (B.L. Larson, ed.). The Iowa State Univ. Press: Ames, Iowa, pp. 164-197.

Kindstedt, P.S., Pell, A.N., Rippe, J.K., Tsang, D.S., and Hartnell, G.F. 1991. Effect of long-term bovine somatotropin (sometribove) treatment on nitrogen (protein) distribution in Jersey milk. J. Dairy Sci., **74**, 72-80.

Kirchgessner, M., Schwab, W., and Muller, H.L. 1989. Effect of bovine growth hormone on energy metabolism of lactating cows in long-term administration. In, Energy Metabolism of Farm Animals. (Y. van der Honing and W.H. Close, eds.). Pudoc Wageningen: Netherlands, pp. 143-146.

Kline, R.M., Smith, H.W., Green, H.B., and Mowrey, D.H. 1987. Determination of bovine somatotropin levels in milk and blood of dairy cattle. Unpublished report AAC8615 dated May 21, 1987, Lilly Research Laboratories, Greenfield, IN.

Lean, I.J., Troutt, H.F., Bruss, M.L., Farver, T.B., Baldwin, R.L., Galland, J.C., Kratzer, D., Holmberg, C.A., and Weaver, L.D. 1991. Postparturient metabolic and production responses in cows previously exposed to long-term treatment with somatotropin. J. Dairy Sci., **74**, 3429-3445.

Lenoir, J. and Schockmel, L.R. 1987. Composition and processing characteristics of milk from cows in the French Clinical Trial. Unpublished report MLL 90311 dated February 2, 1987, Monsanto Agricultural Co., St. Louis, MO.

Leonard, M., Turner, J.D., and Block, E. 1990. Effects of long term somatotropin injection in dairy cows on milk protein profiles. Can. J. Anim. Sci., **70**, 811.

Linn, J.G. 1988. Factors affecting the composition of milk from dairy cows. In, Designing Foods. National Academy of Sciences. National Academy Press: Washington, D.C. pp. 224-241.

Lough, D.S., Muller, L.D., Kensinger, R.S., Sweeney, T.F., and Griel, Jr., L.C. 1988. Effect of added dietary fat and bovine somatotropin on the performance and metabolism of lactating dairy cows. J. Dairy Sci., **71**, 1161-1169.

Lynch, J.M., Barbano, D.M., Bauman, D.E., and Hartnell, G.F. 1988a. Influence of sometribove (recombinant methionyl bovine somatotropin) on the protein and fatty acid composition of milk. J. Dairy Sci., **71**(Suppl. 1), 100(Abstr.).

Lynch, J.M., Barbano, D.M., Bauman, D.E., and Hartnell, G.F. 1989a. Influence of sometribove (recombinant methionyl bovine somatotropin) on thermal properties and cholesterol content of milk fat. J. Dairy Sci., **72**(Suppl. 1), 153(Abstr.).

Lynch, J.M., Barbano, D.M., Bauman, D.E., Houghton, G.E., and Hartnell, G.F. 1989b. Influence of sometribove (recombinant methionyl bovine somatotropin) on milk flavor and starter culture growth in milk. J. Dairy Sci., **72**(Suppl. 1), 187(Abstr.).

Lynch, J.M., Senyk, G.F., Barbano, D.M., Bauman, D.E., and Hartnell, G.F. 1988b. Influence of sometribove (recombinant methionyl bovine somatotropin) on milk lipase and protease activity. J. Dairy Sci., **71**(Suppl. 1), 100(Abstr.).

Marshall, R.T. and Cartledge, M.F. 1989. Sometribove, USAN (recombinant methionyl bovine somatotropin), does not affect clotting time of milk. Cultured Dairy Products Journal **24**, 8.

McGuffey, R.K., Basson, R.P., and Spike, T.E. 1991. Lactation response and body composition of cows receiving somatotropin and three ratios of forage to concentrate. J. Dairy Sci., **74**, 3095-3102.

Mehta, J.M. 1988. In vivo metabolism of BST: Isolation and characterization of a major metabolite from bovine serum. Unpublished report MSL 7632 dated January 1988, Monsanto Agricultural Co., St. Louis, MO.

Malven, P.V., Head, H.H., Collier, R.J. and Buonomo, F.C. 1987. Periparturient changes in secretion and mammary uptake of insulin and in concentrations of insulin and insulin-like growth factors in milk of dairy cows, J. Dairy Sci., **70**, 2254-2265.

Miller, M.A., Hildebrandt, J.R., White, T.C., Hammond, B.G., Madsen, K.S. and Collier, R.J. 1989a. Determinations of IGF-I concentrations in raw, pasteurized, and heat-treated milk, Unpublished report MSL 8673 dated January 3, 1989, Monsanto Agricultural Co., St. Louis, MO.

Miller, M.A., White, T.C., and Collier, R.J. 1989b. Effect of sometribove on plasma and milk IGF-I and IGF-2, Unpublished report dated July 1989, Monsanto Agricultural Co., St. Louis, MO.

NRC. 1989. Nutrient requirements of dairy cattle. Sixth Revised Edition, Update 1989. National Research Council. National Academy Press: Washington, D.C.

Ozimek, L., Wolfe, F., Kennelly, J., Pietucha, S., Pikus, W., and de Boer, G. 1989. The effect of recombinant bovine somatotropin on milk protein distribution during one lactation. J. Dairy Sci., **72**(Suppl. 1), 153(Abstr.).

Pearse, M.J. and Mackinlay, A.G. 1989. Biochemical aspects of syneresis: a review. J. Dairy Sci., **72**, 1401-1407.

Peel, C.J. and Bauman, D.E. 1987. Somatotropin and lactation. J. Dairy Sci., **70**, 474-486.

Pikus, W., Ozimek, L., Wolfe, F., Kennelly, J., and de Boer, G. 1989. The effect of recombinant bovine somatotropin on heat stability of milk and partition of milk salts. J. Dairy Sci., **72** (Suppl. 1), 154(Abstr.).

Rogan, G.J., Mehta, J.M., Janson, C., and Torkelson, A.R. 1988. Isolation of BST metabolites from BST-injected dairy cows by affinity chromatography. Unpublished report MSL 7580 dated April 25, 1988, Monsanto Agricultural Co., St. Louis, MO.

Schams, D., and Karg, H. 1988b. Technical report on BST in dairy cows in 1987. Unpublished Elanco report dated April 19, 1988. Technische Universitat Munchen, Institute of Physiology, D-8050 Freising-Weihenstephan.

Schams, D., and Karg, H. 1988c. Technical report on BST in dairy cows in 1988. Unpublished Elanco report dated September 23, 1988. Technische Universitat Munchen, Institute of Physiology, D-8050 Freising-Weihenstephan.

Schams, D., Karg, H., and Wollny, C. 1988a. Effect of exogenous BST on peripheral blood concentrations of BST and IGF-I in Simmental cows, Unpublished Monsanto Report MLL 90359 dated March 14, 1988, Technische Universitat Munchen, Institute of Physiology, D-8050 Freising-Weihenstephan.

Schingoethe, D.J. and Cleale, R.M. 1989. Effect of stage of lactation, diet composition and daily injections of 10.3 mg BST monomer to mature lactating Holstein cows on concentrations of insulin-like growth factor-I in milk. Unpublished report FD 37-51 dated May 30, 1989, American Cyanamid Company, Princeton, NJ.

Sechen, S.J., Bauman, D.E., Tyrrell, H.F., and Reynolds, P.J. 1989. Effect of somatotropin on kinetics of nonesterified fatty acids and partition of energy, carbon, and nitrogen in lactating cows. J. Dairy Sci., **72**, 59-67.

Smith, H.W., Green, H.B., Cain, T.D., Kline, R.M., and Mowrey, D.H. 1985. Determination of bovine growth hormone residues in milk from cows treated with enterokinase linker bovine somatotropin. Unpublished report AAC8516 dated August 1985, Lilly Research Laboratories, Greenfield, IN.

Soderholm, C.G., Otterby, D.E., Linn, J.G., Ehle, F.R., Wheaton, J.E., Hansen, W.P., and Annexstad, R.J. 1988. Effects of recombinant bovine somatotropin on milk production, body composition, and physiological parameters. J. Dairy Sci., **71**, 355-365.

Torkelson, A.R., Dwyer, K.A., and Rogan, G.J. 1987. Radioimmunoassay of somatotropin in milk from cows administered recombinant bovine somatotropin, Abstract:J. Dairy Sci., **70** (Suppl 1), 146.

Torkelson, A.R., Lanza, G.M., Birmingham, B.K., Vicini, J.L., White, T.C., Dyer, S.E., Madsen, K.S., and Collier, R.J. 1988. Concentrations of insulin-like growth factor 1 (IGF-I) in bovine milk: Effect of herd, stage of lactation, and sometribove, Abstract:J. Dairy Sci., **71**, 152.

Tyrrell, H.F., Brown, A.C.G., Reynolds, P.J., Haaland, G.L., Bauman, D.E., Peel, C.J., and Steinhour, W.D. 1988. Effect of bovine somatotropin on metabolism of lactating dairy cows: energy and nitrogen utilization as determined by respiration calorimetry. J. Nutr., **118**, 1024-1030.

Van den Berg, G. 1989. Milk from rbST-treated cows; its quality and suitability for processing. In, Use of Somatotropin in Livestock Production (K. Sejrsen, M. Vestergaard, and A. Neimann-Sorensen, eds.). Elsevier Science Publishing Co., Inc.: New York, NY. pp. 178-191.

White, T.C., Dyer, S.E., Miller, M.A., Torkelson, A.R., Hudson, S., and Collier, R.J. 1989b. Comparison of milk and plasma concentrations of IGF-I following subcutaneous injections of formulated zinc methionyl bovine growth hormone, Unpublished report MSL 8633 dated January 5, 1989, Monsanto Agricultural Co., St. Louis, MO.

White, T.C., Hildebrandt, J.R., Torkelson, A.R., Miller, M.A., Madsen, K.S., Lanza, G.M., and Collier, R.J. 1989a. Survey of insulin-like growth factor-I (IGF-I) concentrations in commercial bulk tank milk samples, Unpublished report MSL 8671 dated January 10, 1989, Monsanto Agricultural Co., St. Louis, MO.

RACTOPAMINE

IDENTITY

Chemical name: dl-p-α-[[[Hydroxyphenyl-1-methylpropyl] amino]methyl]benzene methanol hydrochloride.

It exists in two diastereomeric forms, which are identified as RS,SR and RR,SS.

Structural formula:

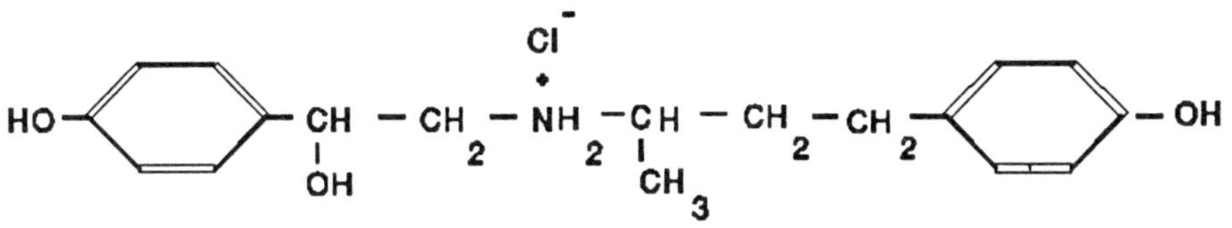

Molecular formula: $C_{18}H_{24}O_3NCl$

Molecular weight: 337.5

OTHER INFORMATION ON IDENTITY AND PROPERTIES

Ractopamine hydrochloride is a phenethanolamine salt which is an off-white to cream coloured solid. It is formulated as a premix containing ractopamine hydrochloride which is then sprayed onto animal feed, usually corn (maize) cob grits, dried and blended.

Melting Point: Not identified

Solubility: Soluble in polar solvents.

RESIDUES IN FOOD AND THEIR EVALUATION

CONDITIONS OF USE

Ractopamine hydrochloride is recommended for continuous feeding to finishing pigs at concentrations of 5 -20 mg/kg for improved feed efficiency and increased rate of live weight gain (LWG). Concentrations of 10-20 mg/kg are recommended for increased carcass leanness and increased carcass dressing percent.

METABOLISM

Pharmacokinetics

Absorption and Bioavailability

The bioavailability of ractopamine hydrochloride was measured in rats and dogs. In both species ractopamine hydrochloride was

- rapidly absorbed into the blood following oral administration
- rapidly cleared from the blood circulation
- mostly associated with the plasma fraction of whole blood

There were large unexplained differences in male and female rats in the absorption and bioabailability of the drug. The results of studies are shown in Table 1.

Table 1. Absorption and bioavailability in rats

Species /Sex	Dose mg/kg	Peak Conc. µg-eq/L	Time to peak (hours)	AUC:Dose Ratio	Half-life (hours)
Rat MA	0.5	0.12	0.5	0.60	
	2.0	0.47	0.5	0.56	6.5
	20.0	3.85	0.5	1.08	14.4
Rat F	0.5	0.16	0.5	0.68	
	2.0	0.81	0.5	0.74	7.5
	20.0	9.02	2.0	3.21	7.5
Dog MA	0.05	0.02	1-2	2.40	
	0.5	0.38	2	3.56	4.0
	5	0.58	2	0.61	6.1
Dog F	0.05	0.02	0.5-2	2.60	
	0.5	0.26	0.5-1	2.72	7.7
	5	0.27	4-8	0.73	7.4

AUC is area under the curve. The values are based on measurements in whole blood. (Data from Elanco submission reports #RO3985, RO4085, RO4185 and DO2385).

Excretion of ractopamine

The excretion of ractopamine after oral dosing was measured in pigs, dogs and monkeys. In all species tested there is a rapid clearance of the drug from the animal with the major route of excretion via the urine. The results of studies are summarised in Table 2.

Table 2. Excretion of ractopamine

Species	Dose	Time (days)	Urine + faeces (%dose)	Urine (%dose)
Dog	0.125 mg/kg	1	>72	majority
		3	79.4	
Monkey	0.125 mg/kg	1	>63	majority
		3	69.8	
Pig	20 mg/kg + 40mg ^{14}C-Ractopamine HCl	1	84.7	82.2
		2	93.1	86.8
		3	95.4	87.6
		7	96.5	88.1

(Data from Elanco report #DO4686, PO3086 and ABC-0330).

METABOLISM

Pigs

The metabolism of ractopamine hydrochloride was studied in pigs fed 30 mg/kg ^{14}C-ractopamine hydrochloride and sacrificed 12 hours after the last dose of the drug. Ractopamine hydrochloride as parent drug is found as a major residue in liver and kidney tissues together with three other key metabolites. The metabolites are three distinct monoglucuronides.

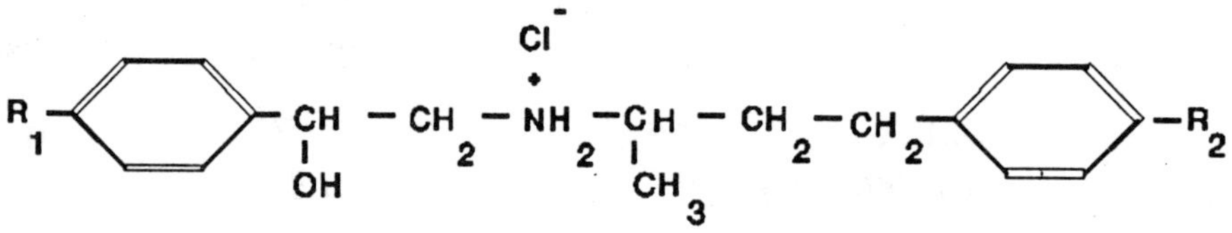

	R1	R2	Isomers
Metabolite A	H	Glucuronide	RS,SR
Metabolite B	H	Glucuronide	RR,SS
Metabolite C	Glucuronide	H	Mixture

The metabolites A and B constitute 30.9% and metabolite C 4.6% of the extractable residues in liver. The extractable residues of the kidney contained 31% of metabolites A and B and 25.9% metabolite C. Similar metabolites are found in liver and kidneys of rats and dogs.

The metabolites were identified by a combination of extraction, enzyme hydrolysis, HPLC, TLC, GC-MS and NMR techniques. (Elanco report #ABC-0355 and later amendment of structures, June, 1992).

Rats and Dogs

One male dog and one female dog were administered by gavage ^{14}C-ractopamine hydrochloride dissolved in water. The dose was 0.5 mg/kg and given 3 times per day for 4 days and once on the fifth day. Samples of urine and faeces were collected . Six hours after the last dose the animals were sacrificed and liver, kidney and bile collected (Elanco report #ABC-0301).

Twelve male and twelve female rats were dosed once daily by gavage with 2 mg/kg ^{14}C-ractopamine hydrochloride for seven days. Each day urine and faeces were collected and liver and kidney tissues collected at slaughter (6 hours after last dose) (Elanco report #ABC-0285).

The samples were analyzed for parent drug and metabolites and the results for dogs, rats and pigs are summarised in Table 3.

Table 3. Metabolic profile in pigs, dogs and rats

	LIVER (mg/kg)			KIDNEY (mg/kg)		
	Pig	Dog	Rat	Pig	Dog	Rat
Parent	0.12	0.59	0.40	0.10	0.50	0.33
Metab A	0.03	0.46	0.17	0.05	0.18	0.52
Metab B	0.04	0.77	0.15	0.06	0.27	0.57
Metab C	0.02	1.76	0.10	0.09	0.63	0.08

TISSUE RESIDUE DEPLETION STUDIES

Radiolabelled Residue Depletion Studies

All of the submitted studies describe radiometric studies in the pig, the species for which the drug is indicated. Several studies are reported and the radiolabel is always carbon-14 positioned either in ring A or ring B. In some studies the radiolabelled drug is a mixture of ractopamine hydrochloride labelled in either ring. The position of the label has no effect on the results since in almost all of the identified residues the parent drug molecule remains intact.

In five of the reported studies the dose is 30 mg/kg in the feed. This is 1.5 times the highest anticipated dose level. The sixth study used 20 mg/kg ractopamine in the feed for seven days.

Study 1. (Elanco Report #ABC-0231).

Three barrows and three gilts were fed 30 ppm ^{14}C-ractopamine hydrochloride for 7 days. The animals were sacrificed at 0.25, 3 and 5 day withdrawal period. The total residues are shown in Table 4.

Table 4. Total residues of ^{14}C-ractopamine hydrochloride (as mg/kg equivalent parent drug) in pigs

	0.25 day	3 days	5 days
Muscle	0.030	0.006	0.002
Kidney	0.738	0.024	0.021
Liver	0.176	0.093	0.045
Fat	0.016	0.006	0.006

Study 2. (Elanco Report #ABC-0368).

Three barrows and three gilts were fed 30 mg/kg ^{14}C-ractopamine hydrochloride for 4 days. The animals were sacrificed at 12 hours after the last dose. The total residues and the residue of parent drug are shown in Table 5.

Table 5. Total residues of ^{14}C-ractopamine hydrochloride (as mg/kg equivalents of parent drug) in pigs

	Concentration Total	(mg/kg) Parent drug	% Parent in Total
Kidney	0.405	0.094	23.4
Liver	0.410	0.111	27.2

Study 3. (Elanco Report #ABC-0273)

Pigs were fed 30 mg/kg ^{14}C-ractopamine hydrochloride for 4, 7 or 10 days. The residues in the tissues collected at the end of each treatment period showed that the total residues had reached a steady state by day 4 in both liver and kidney tissues. Residues in muscle and fat were below the level of reliable detection.

Study 4. (Elanco Report #ABC-0283)

This feeding study is superseded by study 5 which provides more time points under the same experimental conditions.

Study 5. (Elanco Report #ABC-0291)

Six barrows and six gilts were fed 30 mg/kg ^{14}C-ractopamine hydrochloride for 4 days. Groups of three animals of mixed sex were sacrificed at 0.5, 2, 4 and 7 days after the last dose. The total residues are shown in Table 6.

Table 6. Total residues of ^{14}C-ractopamine hydrochloride (mg/kg equivalents parent drug) in pigs

	0.5 day	2 days	4 days	7 days
Muscle	0.02	0.00	0.00	0.00
Kidney	0.60	0.06	0.03	0.02
Liver	0.42	0.10	0.05	0.06
Fat	0.02	0.00	0.00	0.00

Study 6. (Elanco reports T4V739003 and T4V739004)

In this radiolabeled residue depletion study, eight barrows and eight gilts received ^{14}C-ractopamine hydrochloride at 20 mg/kg in the feed for seven days. Three barrows and three gilts were sacrificed after 24 and 48 hour withdrawal periods and two barrows and two gilts were sacriced after a 72 hour withdrawal period. After each sacrifice the ^{14}C-residue concentration was determined in liver, kidney, muscle and fat. The ractopamine (as hydrochloride equivalents) concentration was determined in liver and kidneys. The mean total radioactivity and the mean concentration of ractopamine (as hydrochloride equivalents) calculated as μg/kg of ractopamine in liver and kidney is summarized in Table 7. Muscle and fat did not contain detectable residues at any of the withdrawal periods in this study.

Table 7. Residues of ^{14}C-ractopamine (μg/kg) in pigs fed 20 mg/kg medicated feed

Withdrawal Time (hours)	Liver Total residues	Liver Ractopamine	Kidney Total residues	Kidney Ractopamine
24	106	14.8	116	32.1
48	73	3.7	48	8.3
72	56	1.7	36	3.4

(Ref. Dalidowicz, J.E., Macy, T.D., Cochrane, R.L., Elanco Reports T4V739003 and T4V739004)

The percent ractopamine compared to total residues in liver declined from 14% at 24 hours to 5% at 48 hours and to 3% at 72 hours. Similarly, the percent ractopamine residues in kidney declined from 30% at 24 hours to 17% at 48 hours and to 9% at 72 hours.

All the results for the total residues in liver and kidney tissue are combined in the following two figures. They show a steady log-based decline with a flattening out after 3-4 days. This latter effect is due to the persistence of nonextractable bound residues.

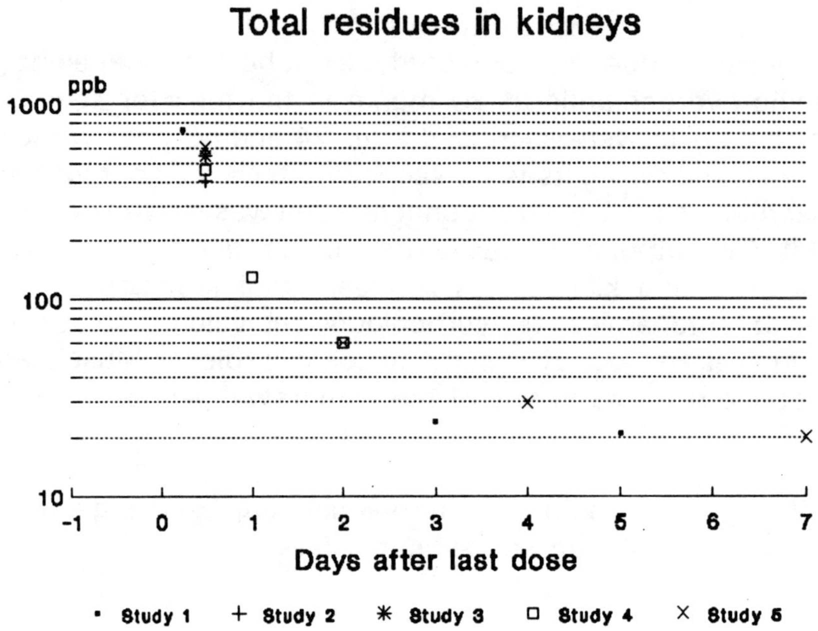
Total residues in kidneys
ppb
1000
100
10
-1
0
1
2
3
4
5
6
7
Days after last dose
Study 1
Study 2
Study 3
Study 4
Study 5

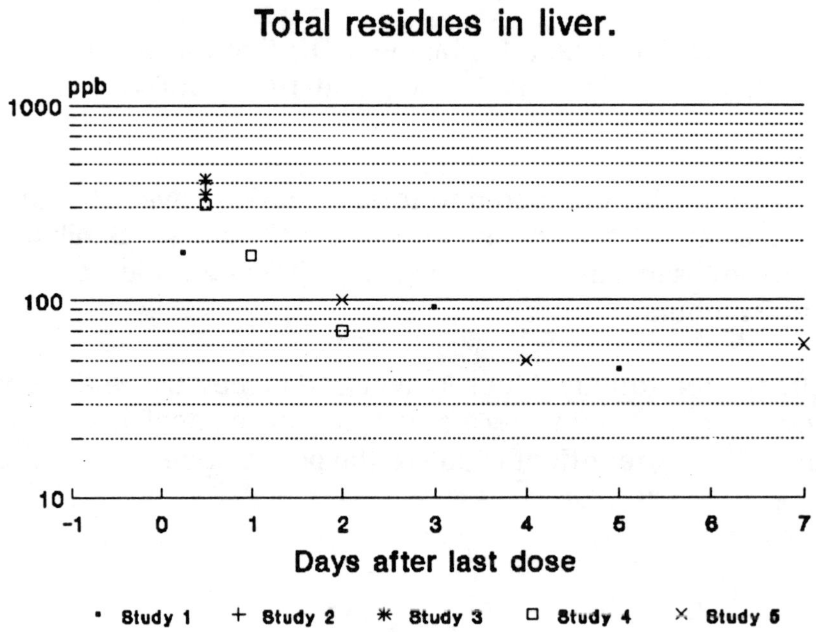
Total residues in liver.
ppb
1000
100
10
-1
0
1
2
3
4
5
6
7
Days after last dose
Study 1
Study 2
Study 3
Study 4
Study 5

OTHER RESIDUE DEPLETION STUDIES

Residue Depletion Studies with Unlabeled Drug

Two studies were carried out by the sponsors using HPLC to measure the residues of parent drug in pigs administered ractopamine-HCl. The HPLC method with electrochemical end-point detection is a validated method which measures the concentration of parent drug in biological samples. The assay does not measure residues of the glucuronide metabolites which are a major fraction of the total residue (see Table 3) since no hydrolysis step is incorporated into the assay. The information would be more meaningful if the parent drug and the ractopamine-glucuronides had been measured. The total of parent drug and it's glucuronide metabolites could have provided information regarding a possible marker residue. There is no firm indication of what percentage of the total residues the parent drug represents because the ratio of parent drug to glucuronides appears to be highly variable.

In another residue depletion study, six pigs were fed 31 mg/kg ractopamine-HCl for seven days. The pigs were sacrificed 12 hours after withdrawal of the drug and the residues of ractopamine-HCl were measured in kidney and liver samples by HPLC. Residues of ractopamine-HCl were 0.058 ± 0.027 mg/kg in liver and 0.118 ± 0.054 mg/kg in kidney.

In a similar study forty eight crossbred pigs were fed ractopamine-HCl at 20 mg/kg for 14 days. Groups of eight pigs (4MA, 4F) were slaughtered at 12 h, 1, 2, 3, 4 and 5 days after drug withdrawal. The residues were measured in the edible tissues by HPLC and the results are shown in Table 8.

Table 8. Residues of ractopamine-HCl in pigs (µg/kg) measured by HPLC

WT (days)	Liver	Kidney	Muscle	Fat	Skin
0.5	11.1	31.8	5.4	<2.0	7.5
1	5.8	12.7	1.9	<1.0	NA
2	3.4	6.7	NA	NA	NA
3	1.7	3.0	NA	NA	NA
4	1.2	2.2	NA	NA	NA
5	NDR	<1.0	NA	NA	NA

NDR is no detectable residue; NA is not analyzed.

The residues measured in pigs given a 31 mg/kg oral dose are 5.2 times higher in liver and 3.7 times higher in kidney than pigs fed 20 mg/kg.

In the most recent study on ractopamine tissue residue depletion in pigs, 30 crossbred pigs were fed 20 mg/kg ractopamine treated ration for nine days. Six pigs, three barrows and three gilts, were sacrificed at one, two, three, four and five days withdrawal. Tissues were collected and subjected to quantitative analysis using HPLC with electrochemical detection. Results are summarized in Table 9.

Table 9. Mean concentration of ractopamine (as HCl equivalents) residue depletion in pig tissue in μg/kg

Withdrawal time (days)	Liver	Kidney
1	11.1	24.6
2	3.2	7.9
3	2.2	2.0
4	1.2	2.3
5	1.4	1.9

(Ref. Tuberg, M.P., Macy, T.D., Cochrane, R.L., Elanco study T4V739001)

Bound Residues and Bioavailability

Pigs were fed 30 mg/kg ^{14}C-ractopamine-HCl for four days. The mean concentration of nonextractable residues, calculated as mg/kg ractopamine-HCl, remaining in the liver and kidney after a one time extraction with 1.0*N* perchloric acid - ethanol (1:1) is summarised in Table 10. The values in parentheses are the non extractable residues as a percentage of the total residues.

Table 10. Nonextractable residues (mg/kg) in pig tissues

Tissue	0.5 d	2 d	4 d	7 d
Liver	0.12 (29%)	0.06 (60%)	0.04 (80%)	0.04 (67%)
Kidney	0.08 (13%)	NA	NA	NA

NA is not assayed

The nature of the nonextractable residues was not fully investigated. The residue pattern is typical of many drugs in that as the total residues in the tissues decrease, the nonextractable portion of the total residues increases.

METHODS OF ANALYSIS FOR RESIDUES IN TISSUES

A method based on HPLC with electrochemical detection is available for the measurement of residues of ractopamine in the edible tissues of pigs. The method measures the concentration of ractopamine as the sum of the four possible stereoisomers. The method is described below.

Ractopamine is extracted from tissues with methanol. Water is added and the extract evaporated down under nitrogen to yield an aqueous extract. The extract is buffered to pH 10.5 with sodium carbonate and the ractopamine extracted with ethyl acetate. The ethyl acetate fraction is further purified on an acid-washed silica cartridge. An aliquot of the purified extract is assayed by HPLC with electrochemical detection.

The method has been carefully validated for

a) linearity of response; standard curve 2 to 300 ng/ml , r = 0.9998

b) precision, reproducibility (interassay CV) in liver and kidney for concentrations 25 to 100 µg/kg was between 2.2 to 3.8%

c) recovery; the recoveries of spikes of ractopamine-HCl at 25, 50 and 100 µg/kg were 77 to 79%

d) specificity; no significant interferences were present in the chromatograms

e) the limit of detection; based on the response from the control tissue (muscle, liver, kidney or fat) at 3 times the signal to noise ratio (SNR) the limit of detection was calculated as 1.5 µg/kg. The sponsors indicate that the sensitivity of the assay has been improved to 0.5 µg/kg (Personal communication to JECFA, June 1992)

f) the limit of quantification based on 10 times the SNR was 5 µg/kg

The method does not measure the ractopamine glucuronides. The sponsors reported some success with kidney tissue but with liver the process required so many clean-up steps that they concluded the method repeatability would be too low (Personal communication to JECFA, June 1992).

APPRAISAL

Ractopamine hydrochloride is specifically indicated for use in the feed of pigs. The highest recommended dose in feed is 20 mg/kg.

The metabolism is similar for the rat, dog and pig. The drug is rapidly absorbed from the gut and is rapidly excreted, mostly via the urine. The major metabolites are the ractopamine glucuronides which together with parent drug account for almost all of the extractable residues.

There is adequate information from six radiometric studies about the total residues in the edible tissues. The highest concentrations are found in the liver and kidney. The total residues decline rapidly after drug withdrawal. This decline over seven days is mostly associated with the extractable residues. The nonextractable residues appear to have a longer half-life.

The parent drug is a significant fraction of the extractable residues, but less than half of the extractable residues are found in liver or kidney at 12 hours after drug withdrawal. The lack of more information on the ratios of parent drug to metabolites in the edible tissues makes it inappropriate to use the parent drug as a marker residue for total residues especially at withdrawal times longer than 24 hours.

The establishment of an MRL will have to consider the total residues because there is no information on the toxicity of the bound residues.

The HPLC assay for parent drug is well validated but it does not measure the extractable glucuronides and therefore may not be appropriate for measuring a marker residue. Determining the acceptability of an analytical method for compliance with the MRL requires consideration of how the HPLC method can be applied or even modified to take into account the metabolites.

ISOMETAMIDIUM

IDENTITY

Chemical names: 3-Amino-8-[3-[3-(aminoiminomethyl)phenyl]-1-triazenyl]-5-ethyl-6-phenylphenanthridinium chloride

8-[3-(m-Amidinophenyl)-2-triazeno]-3-amino-5-ethyl-6-phenylphenanthridinium chloride

7-m-Amidinophenyldiazoamino-2-amino-10-ethyl-9-phenylphenanthridinium chloride

Synonyms: Samorin and Trypamidium

Structural formula:

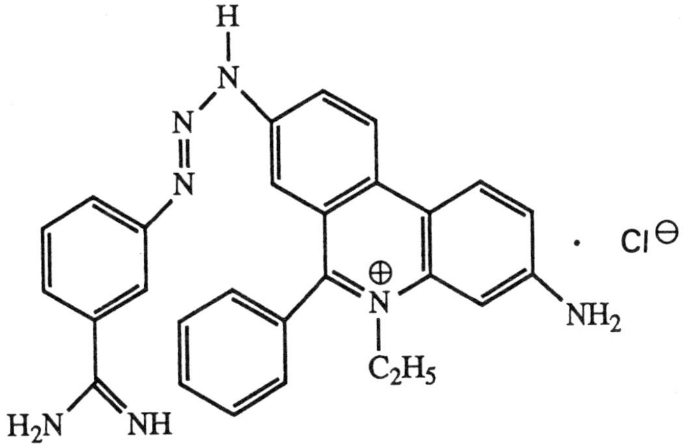

Molecular formula: $C_{28}H_{26}N_7Cl$

Molecular weight: 496.04

OTHER INFORMATION ON IDENTITY AND PROPERTIES

Pure active ingredient

Appearance: Red crystals from aqueous methanol

Melting Point: Decomposes at 244-245°C

Technical Active Ingredients

The commercially available products, Samorin and Trypamidium, have isometamidium chloride as the principle component (~60%) with the remaining fraction comprising of two isomers, two analogs of a bis-species and homidium. Homidium is present at less than 1% and usually 0.5% of the drug. Isometamidium is presented as a dark reddish-brown powder with a solubility in water of 6% (w/v) at 20°C.

RESIDUES IN FOOD AND THEIR EVALUATION

CONDITIONS OF USE

General

Isometamidium is an antitrypanosomal agent. It is used for the treatment and prevention of animal trypanosomiasis principally in cattle but also in sheep, goats, buffalo, donkeys, horses, camels and dogs. Activity has been demonstrated against *Trypanosoma congolense*, *T.vivax*, *T.brucei*, and *T.evansi*. (Touratier, 1981)

The predominant conditions of use are as follows:

In an average infected region: 2 to 4 treatments at 0.5 mg/kg (intramuscular route) every year

In a heavily infected region: 4 to 6 treatments at 0.5 mg/kg (intramuscular route) every year or 2 to 4 treatments at 1 mg/kg (intramuscular route) every year. Concerning this latter dosage, the authors state that in practice it is only used in Republic of Central Africa.

Dosages

Isometamidium is prepared as a 1%, 2% or 4% (w/v) injectable aqueous suspension to be administered intramuscularly at a dose rate of 0.5 or 1.0 mg/kg body weight. Occasionally it is administered by intravenous injection (Dowler et al., in press). For intravenous use in cattle, isometamidium is used as a 1% aqueous solution to be administered at 0.6 mg/kg.

METABOLISM

Pharmacokinetics and bioavailability

The distribution and elimination of isometamidium was examined in lactating dairy cattle following intramuscular injection, 1.0 mg/kg, of ^{14}C-labeled material (Bridge et al, 1982). Peak concentrations of radiolabeled products were detected in plasma at 24 hrs (0.027 μg/ml) post dose and steadily declined to the limit of detection (0.01 μg/ml) by 29 days.

Kinabo and Bogan (1988b) investigated the absorption and distribution of isometamidium and its effect on tissues in cattle following intramuscular injection at 0.5 mg/kg body weight. The drug was rapidly detectable in serum at a mean concentration of only 0.020 µg/ml and declined to concentrations of lower than 0.010 µg/ml within two hours. After 120 hours, serum levels of isometamidium were below the limit of detection.

The distribution of isometamidium was examined in three lactating cows that were administered an IM injection of 1 mg [6-^{14}C]-Samorin/kg body weight in a 2% aqueous solution (Hawkins et al., 1991). Plasma concentrations of radioactivity peaked within 1 hour after dosing (0.051 - 0.160 µg/ml) and then decreased to 0.01 - 0.021 µg/ml at 12 hours. There was no significant decrease in plasma concentrations of radioactivity after 12 hours. The limit of detection was 0.006 µg/ml.

The absorption of ^{14}C-isometamidium was investigated in female rats following a single 1 mg/kg oral dose (Smith et al., 1981). Minimal absorption of the dose was observed. By day 7 after dosing, all tissues contained less than 0.010 mg/kg, at which time 99% of the administered dose had been voided in the feces.

The relay bioavailability of isometamidium residues in bovine tissues was examined in rats. Sixteen adult male rats were fed for 7 and 21 days with a standard diet containing lyophilized liver and kidney from a calf dosed IM with a combination of 45 mg of ^{14}C-isometamidium and 73 mg of cold isometamidium at 1 mg/kg body weight. Intake of ^{14}C-isometamidium in residues through the feed was estimated to be 8.64 µg/rat/day. Another six rats were given a single dose of 2.245 mg of ^{14}C-isometamidium/kg body weight by oral gavage as an aqueous solution. No radioactivity was detected (<0.02 ng ^{14}C-isometamidium residues/g wet tissue) in any of the samples from urine, serum, blood, kidney, liver, spleen, muscle, stomach, and small intestine. Cumulative excretion of radioactivity in feces was 89.85% for the 7 day group, 90.48% for the 21 day group, and 92.69% for the oral gavage group. No statistically significant differences were found between the groups. No clinical or pathological lesions were found. The results indicate that isometamidium residues in tissues are not bioavailable to any significant extent. The authors suggest that the poor bioavailability of the residues may be due to the cationic nature and high affinity binding of the drug to macromolecules. (Kinabo et al., 1989)

Metabolism Studies

Studies with rats (Philips et al., 1967) and cattle (Kinabo and Bogan, 1988b) have indicated that isometamidium metabolites could not be found in the blood. The latter study indicated the injection site was the primary depot for prophylaxis. The presence of active metabolites would have been suspected if isometamidium concentrations at the injection site were as transient and low as those in serum.

Cattle

Samples from three lactating cows that were treated with IM injection of 1 mg [6-^{14}C]-Samorin/kg body weight in a 2% aqueous solution were analyzed for patterns of radiolabelled metabolites using the HPLC procedure as described by Mignot et al. (1991b). Qualitatively, it was shown that compounds in liver, kidney, injection site, plasma, and urine were the same as those present in the parent drug. Metabolic profiles in milk and muscle could not be determined due to low levels of radioactivity. Methodology problems occurred in the analysis of plasma, liver, and kidney. Thirty-one percent of total activity was lost when depositing the plasma sample on the C_{18} cartridge for liquid/solid extraction. For liver and kidney, the first step of total radioactivity extraction was unsuccessful, causing the quantity of total radioactivity injected in the HPLC to be variable and yielding unclear chromatograms. Isometamidium was the main component found in all samples except in liver.

For pooled plasma at 1 hour after treatment, final extraction of total radioactivity was 63.4%. After chromatography, isometamidium represented 47.8% with 38.6% for purple isomer and/or bis-compound, 10.8% for pseudo-isometamidium and 2.7% for unknown metabolites. For pooled urine, at day 2 after treatment, final extraction of total radioactivity was 35.6%. After chromatography, isometamidium represented 71.5% of the chromatogram with 13.9% for purple isomer and/or bis-compound, 7.4% for pseudo-isometamidium and 7.1% for unknown metabolites.

For liver, on days 3, 10, and 30, final extraction of total radioactivity was 54.2%, 42.2%, and 37.0%, respectively. After chromatography, the proportion of isometamidium decreased over time (47.8%, 27.7% and 27.2%) so that by day 30, its level was exceeded by purple isomer. Unknown metabolites represented 24.1%, 33.5%, and 24.6%. For kidney, on days 3, 10, and 30, final extraction of total radioactivity was 49.4%, 41.3%, and 55.8% respectively. After chromatography, the proportion of isometamidium fell with time (38.4%, 36.1%, and 21.7%) while purple isomer and pseudo-isometamidium increased with the latter predominating. Unknown metabolites were less than 12%. For injection site, on day 30, final extraction of total radioactivity was 81.5%. After chromatography, isometamidium represented 73.9% of the chromatogram and unknown metabolites represented 5.1%.

Milk concentrations of radioactivity peaked at Day 2 post-injection for cow 1 (0.0068 μg/ml), at Day 3 for cow 2 and 3 (0.0044 and 0.0062 μg/ml). Cow 3 which was the last animal to be sacrificed had milk concentrations of radioactivity that ranged from 0.0014 - 0.0030 μg/ml from Day 5 to Day 31. Concentrations of radioactivity in tissues were highest at the injection site: 422 mg/kg at 72 hours, 233 mg/kg at 240 hours, and 87 mg/kg at 720 hours with an apparent half-life of approximately 12 days. Liver (maximum 4.60 mg/kg) and kidney (maximum 3.39 mg/kg) had the next highest concentrations. Concentrations of radioactivity in skeletal muscle ranged from 0.012-0.017 mg/kg at different sacrifice times. Table 1 shows a summary of total ^{14}C-residues in each tissue assayed and the amount of unchanged isometamidium. (Mignot et al., 1991a; Hawkins et al., 1991)

Table 1. Concentration (mg/kg) of Total Residue (TR) and Unchanged Isometamidium (I) in Tissues of Dairy Cows Treated with 1 mg/kg ^{14}C-Samorin Intramuscularly

Withdrawal	Liver		Kidney		Muscle*	Fat*	Inj. Site	
Time (days)	TR	I	TR	I	TR	TR	TR	I
3	4.72	1.22	3.38	0.64	0.013	0.017	422	NA
10	2.53	0.30	2.53	0.38	0.017	0.007	233	NA
30	2.26	0.23	2.02	0.24	0.012	0.011	96	58

* - Unchanged isometamidium was not determined in these tissues.
NA - Not Analyzed

Rat

Metabolism in rat plasma was determined by dosing thirty-eight female rats with 2 mg/kg Trypamidium by IV. Blood was sampled at 10 and 30 minutes, and 2, 5, 20 and 24 hours after treatment. Another 126 female rats received either 12.5, 50 or 200 mg/kg/day for 21 days by oral gavage. Blood samples were drawn at 30 minutes and 3 hours after treatments on days 0, 13 and 20. After a solid/liquid extraction, plasma extracts were analyzed by HPLC with UV detection. The limit of quantification was 0.01 μg/ml. Following the single IV dose, isometamidium was only measurable at time 10 minutes (0.1772 μg/ml) and 30 minutes (0.0862 μg/ml) after treatment. These results indicate that the rate of elimination is very high. Following the 21 day oral dose, isometamidium could not be detected even at the highest dosage. (Mignot and Lefebvre, 1991)

TISSUE RESIDUE DEPLETION STUDIES

Cattle

In the pharmacokinetic study described previously, Bridge et al. (1982) found the highest concentration of radiolabeled products, 73.5 mg/kg, was located at the injection site 72 hours post-injection. The half-life of the injection site residues was calculated to be 39 days. The liver and kidney tissues were the other main sites of radioactivity localization. The peak concentrations of isometamidium equivalents were 7.1 and 5.8 mg/kg at 72 hours with elimination half-lives of 25 and 35 days for the liver and kidney tissues respectively. In addition to tissues, milk samples were collected and analyzed during the 90 day post injection period. Most of the samples had levels of isometamidium which were below the limit of detection (0.01 μg/ml). However, some cows did produce positive samples (0.0138 - 0.0174 μg/ml) on single occasions from 5 to 70 days post-injection.

Isometamidium residues in calves have been reported using a sensitive HPLC method. In this study the calves were administered isometamidium at 0.5 mg/kg by IM injection. Isometamidium was only detectable in the serum up to 2 hours after injection, at a mean maximum concentration of 0.02 μg/ml. The highest concentration of isometamidium was detected at the injection site at 7, 21 and 42 days. The results of the various tissue assays have been tabulated in Table 2. (Kinabo and Bogan, 1988b)

Table 2. Isometamidium Residues in Calf Tissues (mg/kg) in Mean ± SD after IM Injection of 0.5 mg/kg

Tissue	Days Post-injection 7	21	42
Injection site	1270 ± 272	315 ± 173	208 ± 94
Liver	4.80 ± 0.84	4.07 ± 0.35	0.75 ± 1.41
Kidney	5.21 ± 3.36	2.98 ± 0.64	0.70 ± 0.11
Muscle	1.00 ± 0.02	0.87 ± 0.01	0.59 ± 0.12

Isometamidium residues were determined by treating 19 young bulls with a single gluteal IM injection of 1 mg/kg. Blood samples were drawn 10 times between 0.25 and 48 hours after dosing, on days 3, 5, 9, and at approximately weekly intervals until sacrifice. Tissue samples were collected at 1, 3, and 6 months after treatment. Samples were analyzed using the method of Mignot et al. (1991b). For bulls slaughtered one month post-treatment, the plasma concentration of isometamidium (mean = 30.82 ng/ml) peaked at one hour post-dosing. Levels declined rapidly thereafter so that in two out of five animals at 48 hours and in five out of five at 72 hours, they were below the limit of quantification (0.008 μg/ml). Isometamidium levels in muscle and fat from all animals were below the limit of quantification at all sacrifice times (0.1 mg/kg). In liver, the mean concentration of isometamidium was 0.251 mg/kg at one month post-treatment. At three months post-treatment, isometamidium was detected in only one out of five livers (0.132 mg/kg). At six months post-treatment, no isometamidium was detected in any of the livers. In kidney at one month post-treatment, isometamidium was detected in all animals. At three and six months post-treatment, no isometamidium was detected in any kidney. At the injection site one month post-treatment, mean isometamidium concentration was 129.5 mg/kg. By 3 months, the mean level dropped to 38.7 mg/kg. At 6 months, the mean level was 1.35 mg/kg and two bulls had values below the limit of quantification. Table 3 shows the concentrations of isometamidium in bull tissues at 1, 3, and 6 months following a single injection. (Mignot et al., 1991c; Bosc et al., 1991)

Table 3. Isometamidium Concentrations (mg/kg) in Mean ± SD after IM Injection of 1 mg/kg in Young Bulls

Withdrawal Time (months)	Fat	Muscle	Liver	Kidney	Inj. Site
1	BQ	BQ	0.251 ± 0.03	0.386 ± 0.13	129.5 ± 145.9
3	BQ	BQ	BQ	BQ	38.7 ± 37.7
6	BQ	BQ	BQ	BQ	1.346 ± 0.7

BQ: Below the limit of quantification (0.1 μg/ml)

Goats

Isometamidium residues in goats treated by intramuscular and intravenous injection at a level of 0.5 mg/kg were evaluated using a spectrophotometric method (Braide and Eghianruwa, 1980). Table 4 shows the concentrations of isometamidium found in tissues 4 and 12 weeks after a single dose.

Table 4. Isometamidium Residues (mg/kg) in Goat Tissues

Tissue	Time (weeks)	Route of Administration Intramuscular	Intravenous
Liver	4	5.52 ± 0.38	11.39 ± 0.61
	12	ND	6.78 ± 0.29
Kidney	4	2.51 ± 0.16	9.29 ± 0.52
	12	<1.25	3.26 ± 0.20
Muscle	4	ND	ND
	12	NA	NA
Fat	4	ND	ND
	12	NA	NA
Injection Site	4	2.51 ± 0.21	ND
	12	ND	NA

ND - Not detected

METHODS OF ANALYSIS FOR RESIDUES IN TISSUES

Earlier analytical procedures lacked sensitivity and specificity such as the spectrophotometric method (Philips et al., 1967) which could not detect isometamidium concentrations less that 1 µg/ml in the plasma. The HPLC method developed by Perschke and Vollner (1985) was indirect in that isometamidium was converted to homidium before assay and therefore not specific.

Most of the methods reported for isometamidium, or isometamidium isomers and analogues, are for determination in plasma or serum. Kinabo and Bogan (1988a) developed an analytical procedure using solid-phase extraction and ion-pair reverse phase HPLC with fluorescence detection for isometamidium in bovine serum and tissues. Although the assay could detect levels of isometamidium down to 0.010 µg/ml in serum, the sensitivity was limited to 0.50 mg/kg in the tissue. The authors suggest that this may be due to strong binding of isometamidium to mucopolysaccharides, nucleic acid and lipids.

An improved method to assay isometamidium in body fluids and tissues has been developed (Mignot et al., 1991c). Isometamidium is separated from endogenous compounds with a C_{18} cartridge (solid-liquid extraction) and the sample is injected into an HPLC. The method is capable of separating isometamidium from other Trypamidium compounds. In this study, only isometamidium was measured quantitatively. The percent recoveries from fortified matrices were as follows: plasma 76%, fat 68%, kidney 68%, muscle 61%, liver 56%, milk 89%, and urine 89%. The calibration curves are linear for concentrations ranging from 0 to 160 ng/ml for plasma and from 0 to 1000 ng/ml (or µg/kg) for milk and tissues. The limits of quantification are 8 ng/ml for plasma, 10 ng/ml for urine, and 100 µg/kg (or ng/ml) for fat, muscle, kidney, liver, and milk. Specificity was demonstrated by the lack of chromatographic peaks from interfering biological compounds.

APPRAISAL

An evaluation of new residue data for isometamidium has been completed. In the metabolism study in lactating cows injected with ^{14}C-Samorin, it was shown qualitatively that the metabolites found in plasma, urine, injection site, liver and kidney were the same as those present in the parent drug but no homidium was detected. Metabolic profiles in milk and muscle could not be determined due to low levels of radioactivity. Isometamidium was the main component found in kidney and the injection site, but not liver. It was determined that parent isometamidium comprises only 20 and 16% of the total residue in liver and kidney.

The bioavailability of isometamidium residues was measured by refeeding lyophilized calf tissues containing incurred residues of ^{14}C-Samorin to rats and measuring the amount of radioactivity absorbed and excreted by the rats. The results of this assessment showed that there were no detectable residues in the urine, serum, blood, kidney, liver, spleen, muscle, stomach, or small intestine of the rats. Cumulative excretion of radioactivity in the rat feces was approximately 90% after oral dosing with calf tissues containing incurred isometamidium residues and 93% after oral dosing of drug in an aqueous solution. The results indicate that isometamidium residues in tissues are not bioavailable to any significant extent. The poor bioavailability of the residues may be due to the cationic nature and high affinity binding of the drug to macromolecules.

In the study of isometamidium residues in young bulls, plasma levels dropped to below the limit of quantification by 72 hours after treatment. Tissue samples were collected at 1, 3, and 6 months after treatment. Muscle and fat had isometamidium levels that were below the limit of quantification at all three sacrifice times. At three months post-treatment, isometamidium was detected in only one out of five livers. At six months post-treatment, no isometamidium was detected in any of the livers. By three months, isometamidium concentration in kidney had dropped below the limit of quantification. At six months, two out of five injection sites had isometamidium levels below the limit of quantification.

In lactating cows, isometamidium levels in milk peaked on day 2 (6.8 µg/L) and remained below 3 µg/L after day 7.

An improved HPLC method for measuring isometamidium residues in milk and tissue has been developed. The sponsor has validated the method to 0.1 mg/kg, and the percent recoveries, linearity, intraday precision and accuracy, and limit of quantification reported are acceptable.

Based on the ADI of 0-100 µg/kg established by JECFA, the permitted daily intake of isometamidium would be 6 mg of total drug-related residue contributed by 500 g of food animal meat plus 1.5 L of the milk in the diet of a 60-kg person. At 30 days of withdrawal, the intake of residues of isometamidium is well below the ADI. Based on the data from the study in bulls administered isometamidium at 1 mg/kg intramuscularly, JECFA recommended an MRL of 100 µg/kg for parent isometamidium in muscle and fat, 500 µg/kg in liver, 1000 µg/kg in kidney, and 100 µg/L in milk (see Table 5).

Table 5. Recommended MRLs for Isometamidium in Cattle

Tissue	Concentration at Day 30 Withdrawal, mg/kg 1 mg/kg IM	Total Residue Consumed mg(a)	Recommended MRL µg/kg parent	Theoretical Maximum Daily Intake mg(a)
Muscle	<0.1	0.03	100	0.03
Liver	0.25(1.25)b	0.12	500(2500)b	0.25
Kidney	0.39(2.44)c	0.12	1000(6300)c	0.31
Fat	<0.1	0.01	100	0.01
Milk	0.0068(d)	0.01	100(e)	0.15
Total		0.29		0.75

a) Based on a daily intake of 0.3 kg muscle, 0.1 kg liver, 0.05 kg kidney and fat, and 1.5 L milk
b) Adjusted observed value by 20% to estimate total residues
c) Adjusted observed value by 16% to estimate total residues
d) This value represents the highest concentration of total isometamidium residues found in milk. It occurs 2 days after dosing
e) This MRL µg/L in milk is based on the limit of quantitation of the analytical method

The injection site concentrations at 30 days withdrawal averaged 96 mg/kg; however, it was determined that this does not adversely impact human food safety for the following reasons:

1) isometamidium residues in tissues are not bioavailable to any significant extent,
2) consumption of an injection site would be extremely rare, and
3) the maximum theoretical intake of residues from muscle, liver, kidney, fat and milk of isometamidium at 30 days withdrawal is well below the ADI.

REFERENCES

Bosc, F., Huet, A.M., Aumont, D., Bernardin, J.B., Longo, F., Rolland, M.L. and Weil, A. 1991. Determination of isometamidium concentrations in plasma and tissue samples of young bulls following intramuscular administration of trypamidium at a level of 1 mg/kg (Animal Phase). Unpublished report submitted to FAO by Rhone Merieux, Toulouse Cedex, France.

Braide, V. and Eghianruwa, K.I. 1980. Isometamidium Residues in Goat Tissues after Parenteral Administration. Res. Vet. Sci., **29**, 111-113.

Bridge, C.M., Smith, G.E., Smith, R., Templeton, R. and Yoxall, A.T. 1982. Samorin: Study in the lactating cow, of the distribution and excretion of radiolabelled drug-derived products, following the administration of a single intramuscular dose of [6-14C] Samorin. M & B Research Report R. Ph. 176.

Dowler, M.B.E., Schillinger, D. and Connor, R.J. (in press). Notes on the routine intravenous use of isometamidium in the control of bovine trypanosomiasis in the Kenya Coast. Trop Anim. Hlth Prod.

Hawkins, D.R., Elsom, L.F., Kane, T.J. and Cameron, D.M. 1991. The pharmacokinetics and metabolism of ^{14}C-Samorin in lactating cows. Unpublished report submitted to FAO by Rhone Merieux, Toulouse Cedex, France.

Kinabo, L.D.B. and Bogan, J.A. 1988a. Solid-phase extraction and ion-pair reversed-phase HPLC of isometamidium bovine serum and tissues. Acta Trop. (in press).

Kinabo, L.D.B. and Bogan, J.A. 1988b. Pharmacokinetic and histopathological investigation of isometamidium in cattle. Res. Vet. Sci., **44**, 267-269.

Kinabo, L.D.B., Bogan, J.A., McKellar, Q.A. and Murray, M. 1989. Relay bioavailability and toxicity of isometamidium residues: a model for human risk assessment. Vet. Hum. Tox., **31**, 417-421.

Mignot, A. and Lefebvre, M. 1991. Determination of isometamidium concentrations in plasma of rats after IV administration (2 $mg \cdot kg^{-1}$) and repeated oral administrations (12.5, 50, 200 $mg \cdot kg^{-1} \cdot day^{-1)}$. Unpublished report submitted to FAO by Rhone Merieux, Toulouse Cedex, France.

Mignot, A., Lefebvre, M., Couerbe, P. and Vidal, R. 1991a. Study on the Metabolism following single intramuscular administration of ^{14}C-Samorin (1 $mg \cdot kg^{-1}$) to lactating cows. Unpublished report submitted to FAO by Rhone Merieux, Toulouse Cedex, France.

Mignot, A., Lefebvre, M. and Vidal, R. 1991b. Development and validation of a new high-performance liquid chromatography assay of isometamidium. Unpublished report submitted to FAO by Rhone Merieux, Toulouse Cedex, France.

Mignot, A., Lefebvre, M. and Vidal, R. 1991c. Determination of isometamidium concentration in plasma and tissue samples of young bulls after an intramuscular administration of trypamidium at a level of 1 $mg \cdot kg^{-1}$. Unpublished report submitted to FAO by Rhone Merieux, Toulouse Cedex, France.

Persche, M. and Vollner, L. 1985. Determination of the trypanocidal drugs Homidium, Isometamidium and Quinapyramine in bovine serum or plasma using HPLC. Acta Trop., **42**, 209-216.

Phillips, F.S., Sternberg, S.S., Cronin, A.P., Sodergen, J.E. and Vidal, P.M. 1967. Physiological disposition and intracellular localization of isometamidium. Cancer Research, **27**(1), 333-349.

Smith, J., Bridge, C.M. and Smith, G.E. 1981. Samorin: Study, in the female rat, of the distribution and excretion of radiolabelled drug-derived products after intramuscular or oral administration of a single dose of [6-14C] Samorin. M & B Research Report RES/3851.

Touratier, L. 1981. (The advantage of using isometamidium for the control at animal trypanosomiasis). International Scientific Council for Trypanosomiasis Research and Control. 16th Meeting, Yaounde, Cameroon, 1979. OAU/STRC. 308-316.

ANNEX 1

SUMMARY OF JECFA EVALUATIONS OF VETERINARY DRUG RESIDUES FROM THE 32ND MEETING TO THE PRESENT

The attached table summarizes the veterinary drug evaluations conducted by JECFA at the 32nd (1987), the 34th (1989), the 36th 91990), the 38th (1991) and the 40th (1992) Meetings. These meetings were devoted exclusively to the evaluation of veterinary drug residues in foods. Please see the Reports for those meetings.

Some notes regarding the table:

- The "Status" column refers to the ADI and indicates if "No" ADI was established, if a "full" ADI was given, or if the ADI is Temporary (TE).
- Where an MRL is temporary, it is so indicated by "TE".
- Several compounds have been evaluated more than once. The data given is for the most recent evaluation.
- The residue on which the MRL is based is <u>not given</u> and <u>should be obtained</u> from the Reports for the individual meetings. Residues used to calculated MRLs include parent drug, a metabolite, a marker compound and total drug-related residue.

Substance	ADI µg/kg BW	Status	JECFA	MRL µg/kg	Tissue
Chloramphenicol	None	No	32 (1987)	No MRL	
Estradiol 17 ß	Unnecessary	Full	32 (1987)	Unnecessary	Bovine
Progesterone	Unnecessary	Full	32 (1987)	Unnecessary	Bovine
Testosterone	Unnecessary	Full	32 (1987)	Unnecessary	Bovine
Zeranol	0-500	Full	32 (1987)	2	Bovine muscle
				10	Bovine liver
Albendazole	0-50	Full	34 (1989)	100	Muscle, fat, milk
				5000	Liver, kidney
Dimetridazole	None	No	34 (1989)	No MRL	
Diminazene	None	No	34 (1989)	No MRL	
Ipronidazole	None	No	34 (1989)	No MRL	
Metronidazole	None	No	34 (1989)	No MRL	
Ronidazole	0-25	TE	34 (1989)	No MRL	
Sulfadimidine	0-4	Full	38 (1991)	50	Milk
				300	Meat, liver, kidney, fat
Sulphthiazole	None	No	34 (1989)	No MRL	

Substance	ADI µg/kg BW	Status	JECFA	MRL µg/kg	Tissue
Trenbolone acetate	0-0.02	Full	34 (1989)	10	Liver
				2	Muscle
Benzyl penicillin	30	Full	36 (1990)	50	Liver, kidney, muscle
				4	Milk
Carbadox	Limited acceptance	Full	36 (1990)	30	Swine liver
				5	Swine muscle
Levamisole	0-3	TE	36 (1990)	10 (TE)	Edible tissues, milk
Olaquindox	Limited acceptance	Full	36 (1990)	No MRL	
Oxytetracycline	0-3	Full	36 (1990)	100	Muscle
				100	Milk
				10	Fat
				300	Liver
				600	Kidney
				200	Eggs
Carazolol	0-0.1	TE	38 (1991)	5	Muscle, fat (cattle, pigs)
				30	Liver, kidney (cattle, pigs)

Substance	ADI µg/kg BW	Status	JECFA	MRL µg/kg	Tissue
Febantel	0-10	TE	38 (1991)	Group MRL 100	Muscle, fat, kidney (cattle, sheep, pigs)
Fenbendazole	0-25	TE	38 (1991)	Group MRL 500	Liver (cattle, sheep, pigs)
Oxfendazole	0-4	TE	38 (1991)	Group MRL 100	Milk (cattle)
Spiramycin	0-5	TE	38 (1991)	50	Muscle (cattle, pigs)
				300	Liver (cattle, pigs)
				200	Kidney (cattle, pigs)
				150	Milk (cattle)
Tylosin	None	No	38 (1991)	No MRL	
Azaperone	None	No	38 (1991)	No MRL	
Chlorpromazine	None	No	38 (1991)	No MRL	
Propionylpromazine	None	No	38 (1991)	No MRL	
Closantel	0-30	Full	36 (1990)		
			40 (1992)	1000	Muscle, liver (cattle)
				3000	Kidney, fat (cattle)
				1500	Muscle, liver (sheep)
				5000	Kidney (sheep)
				2000	Fat (sheep)

Substance	ADI µg/kg BW	Status	JECFA	MRL µg/kg	Tissue
Flubendazole	0-12	Full	40 (1992)	10	Muscle, Liver (pigs)
				200	Muscle (poultry)
				500	Liver (poultry)
				400	Eggs
Ivermectin	0-1	Full	36 (1990)	15	Liver (other species)
				20	Fat (other species)
			40 (1992)	100	Liver (cattle)
				40	Fat (cattle)
Thiabendazole	0-100	Full	40 (1992)	100	Edible tissues (cattle, pigs, goats, sheep) and milk (cattle, goats)
Triclabendazole	0-3	Full	40 (1992)	200	Muscle (cattle)
				300	Liver, kidney (cattle)
				100	Fat (cattle)
				100	Edible tissues (sheep)
Furazolidone	None	No	40 (1992)	No MRL	
Nirofurazone	None	No	40 (1992)	No MRL	
Bovine Somatotropins	Not specified	Full	40 (1992)	Not specified	Milk, edible tissues (cattle)

Substance	ADI µg/kg BW	Status	JECFA	MRL µg/kg	Tissue
Ractopamine	None	No	40 (1992)	No MRL	
Isometamidium	0-100	Full	40 (1992)	100	Muscle, fat, milk (cattle)
				500	Liver (cattle)
				1000	Kidney (cattle)

ANNEX 2

RECOMMENDATIONS ON COMPOUNDS

Substance	Acceptable Daily Intake (ADI) for humans and other toxicological recommendations	Recommended Maximum Residue Limit (MRL)
Anthelmintic Agents		
Closantel	Not evaluated[1]	Muscle and liver (sheep): 1500 μg/kg[2] Kidney (sheep): 5000 μg/kg[2] Fat (sheep): 2000 μg/kg[2] Muscle and liver (cattle): 1000 μg/kg[2] Kidney and fat (cattle): 3000 μg/kg[2]
Flubendazole	0-12 μg per kg of body weight	Muscle and liver (pigs): 10 μg/kg[2] Muscle (poultry): 200 μg/kg[2] Liver (poultry): 500 μg/kg[2] Eggs: 400 μg/kg[2]
Ivermectin	0-1 μg per kg of body weight	Liver (cattle): 100 μg/kg[3] Fat (cattle): 40 μg/kg[3]
Thiabendazole	0-100 μg per kg of body weight	Edible tissues[4] (cattle, pigs, goats, and sheep) and milk (cattle and goats): 100 μg/kg[5]
Triclabendazole	0-3 μg per kg of body weight	Muscle (cattle): 200 μg/kg[6] Liver and kidney (cattle): 300 μg/kg[6] Fat (cattle): 100 μg/kg[6] Edible tissues[4] (sheep): 100 μg/kg[6]

Antimicrobial Agents		
Furazolidone	Not allocated[7]	No MRLs allocated[8]
Nitrofurazone	Not allocated[9]	No MRLs allocated[8]
Production aids		
Bovine somatotropins	Not specified[10]	Milk and edible tissues[4] (cattle): Not specified[11]
Ractopamine	Not allocated[12]	No MRLs allocated[13]
Trypanocide		
Isometamidium	0-100 μg per kg of body weight	Muscle, fat, and milk (cattle): 100 μg/kg[2] Liver (cattle): 500 μg/kg[2] Kidney (cattle): 1000 μg/kg[2]

1 An ADI of 0-30 μg per kg of body weight was established at the thirty-sixth meeting of the Committee (WHO Technical Report series 799, 1990).

2 Expressed as parent drug.

3 Expressed as 22,23-dihydroavermectin $B_{1a}(H_2B_{1a})$.

4 Edible tissues are defined as muscle, fat, liver, and kidney.

5 Expressed as the sum of thiabendazole and 5-hydroxythiabendazole.

6 Expressed as 5-chloro-6-(2′,3′-dichlorophenoxy)-benzimidazole-2-one.

7 An ADI could not be established because of evidence of genotoxicity and carcinogenicity and lack of information on the nature of the metabolites.

8 MRLs were not allocated because:

a. No ADI was established;
b. Data on residues were not sufficient to identify a marker residue; and
c. Insufficient information was available on the quantity and nature of the total residues.

9 An ADI could not be established because no-effect levels were not observed for the tumorigenic effects.

10 The ADI applies to somagrebove, sometribove, somavubove, and somidobove. ADI "not specified" is a term applicable to a veterinary drug for which there is a large margin of safety for the consumption of its residues based on available toxicity and intake data when the drug is used according to good practice in the use of veterinary drugs. For that reason, and for reasons stated in the individual evaluation, the Committee has concluded that use of the veterinary drug does not represent a hazard to human health and that there is no need to specify a numerical acceptable daily intake.

11 The MRLs apply to somagrebove, sometribove, somavubove, and somidobove. MRL "not specified" is a term applicable to a veterinary drug for which there is a large margin of safety for the consumption of its residues based on available data on the identity and concentration of the residues in animal tissues when the drug is used according to good practice in the use of veterinary drugs. For that reason, and for the reasons stated in the individual evaluation, the Committee has concluded that the presence of drug residues in the indicated animal product does not present a health concern and that there is no need to specify a numerical maximum residue limit.

12 An ADI could not be established because a clear no-effect level was not observed for pharmacological effects and the issue of carcinogenicity has not been resolved.

13 MRLs were not allocated because:

a. An ADI was not established; and
b. Sufficient information was not available to firmly establish a residue marker in animal tissues.

ANNEX 3

RESIDUES OF SOME VETERINARY DRUGS IN ANIMALS AND FOODS
FAO FOOD AND NUTRITION PAPER 41/3, FAO, ROME 1991

CORRIGENDA

Page 11, line 17

Delete > 40 g/kg in muscle ... > 40 g/L in urine.	Insert	> 40 µg/kg in muscle ... > 40 µg/L in urine.

Page 11, line 20

Delete 40 g/kg	Insert	40 µg/kg

Page 11, line 35

Delete 50 g/kg	Insert	50 µg/kg

Page 11, line 38

Delete 54, 60 and 62 g/kg	Insert	54, 60 and 62 µg/kg

Page 12, line 11

Delete 50 g/kg 10 g/L	Insert	50 µg/kg 10 µg/L

Page 12, line 23

Delete g/L	Insert	µg/L

Page 13, line 8

Delete (in g/litre)	Insert	(in µg/litre)

Page 13, line 28

Delete 30-60 g/kg	Insert	30-60 µg/kg

Page 13, line 29

Delete 12.5 g/kg	Insert	12.5 µg/kg

Page 14, line 3

Delete (g/kg)	Insert	(µg/kg)

Page 14, line 33

Delete 10-50 g per litre 50-100 g per kg	Insert	10-50 µg per litre 50-100 µg per kg

FAO TECHNICAL PAPERS

FAO FOOD AND NUTRITION PAPERS

1/1 Review of food consumption surveys 1977 – Vol. 1. Europe, North America, Oceania, 1977 (E)
1/2 Review of food consumption surveys 1977 – Vol. 2. Africa, Latin America, Near East, Far East, 1979 (E)
2 Report of the joint FAO/WHO/UNEP conference on mycotoxins, 1977 (E F S)
3 Report of a joint FAO/WHO expert consultation on dietary fats and oils in human nutrition, 1977 (E F S)
4 JECFA specifications for identity and purity of thickening agents, anticaking agents, antimicrobials, antioxidants and emulsifiers, 1978 (E)
5 JECFA – guide to specifications, 1978 (E F)
5 Rev. 1. JECFA – guide to specifications, 1983 (E F)
5 Rev. 2. JECFA – guide to specifications, 1991 (E)
6 The feeding of workers in developing countries, 1976 (E S)
7 JECFA specifications for identity and purity of food colours, enzyme preparations and other food additives, 1978 (E F)
8 Women in food production, food handling and nutrition, 1979 (E F S)
9 Arsenic and tin in foods: reviews of commonly used methods of analysis, 1979 (E)
10 Prevention of mycotoxins, 1979 (E F S)
11 The economic value of breast-feeding, 1979 (E F)
12 JECFA specifications for identity and purity of food colours, flavouring agents and other food additives, 1979 (E F)
13 Perspective on mycotoxins, 1979 (E F S)
Manuals of food quality control:
14/1 Food control laboratory, 1979 (Ar E)
14/1 Rev. 1. The food control laboratory, 1986 (E)
14/2 Additives, contaminants, techniques, 1980 (E)
14/3 Commodities, 1979 (E)
14/4 Microbiological analysis, 1979 (E F S)
14/5 Food inspection, 1981 (Ar E) (Rev. 1984, E S)
14/6 Food for export, 1979 (E S)
14/6 Rev. 1. Food for export, 1990 (E S)
14/7 Food analysis: general techniques, additives, contaminants and composition, 1986 (C E)
14/8 Food analysis: quality, adulteration and tests of identity, 1986 (E)
14/9 Introduction to food sampling, 1988 (Ar C E F S)
14/10 Training in mycotoxins analysis, 1990 (E S)
14/11 Management of food control programmes, 1991 (E)
14/12 Quality assurance in the food control microbiological laboratory, 1991 (E)
15 Carbohydrates in human nutrition, 1980 (E F S)
16 Analysis of food consumption survey data for developing countries, 1980 (E F S)
17 JECFA specifications for identity and purity of sweetening agents, emulsifying agents, flavouring agents and other food additives, 1980 (E F)
18 Bibliography of food consumption surveys, 1981 (E)
18 Rev. 1. Bibliography of food consumption surveys, 1984 (E)
18 Rev. 2. Bibliography of food consumption surveys, 1987 (E)
18 Rev. 3. Bibliography of food consumption surveys, 1990 (E)
19 JECFA specifications for identity and purity of carrier solvents, emulsifiers and stabilizers, enzyme preparations, flavouring agents, food colours, sweetening agents and other food additives, 1981 (E F)
20 Legumes in human nutrition, 1982 (E F S)
21 Mycotoxin surveillance – a guideline, 1982 (E)
22 Guidelines for agricultural training curricula in Africa, 1982 (E F)
23 Management of group feeding programmes, 1982 (E F P S)
24 Evaluation of nutrition interventions, 1982 (E)
25 JECFA specifications for identity and purity of buffering agents, salts; emulsifiers, thickening agents, stabilizers; flavouring agents, food colours, sweetening agents and miscellaneous food additives, 1982 (E F)
26 Food composition tables for the Near East, 1983 (E)
27 Review of food consumption surveys 1981, 1983 (E)
28 JECFA specifications for identity and purity of buffering agents, salts, emulsifiers, stabilizers, thickening agents, extraction solvents, flavouring agents, sweetening agents and miscellaneous food additives, 1983 (E F)
29 Post-harvest losses in quality of food grains, 1983 (E F)
30 FAO/WHO food additives data system, 1984 (E)
30 Rev. 1. FAO/WHO food additives data system, 1985 (E)
31/1 JECFA specifications for identity and purity of food colours, 1984 (E F)
31/2 JECFA specifications for identity and purity of food additives, 1984 (E F)
32 Residues of veterinary drugs in foods, 1985 (E/F/S)
33 Nutritional implications of food aid: an annotated bibliography, 1985 (E)
34 JECFA specifications for identity and purity of certain food additives, 1986 (E F**)
35 Review of food consumption surveys 1985, 1986 (E)
36 Guidelines for can manufacturers and food canners, 1986 (E)
37 JECFA specifications for identity and purity of certain food additives, 1986 (E F)
38 JECFA specifications for identity and purity of certain food additives, 1988 (E)
39 Quality control in fruit and vegetable processing, 1988 (E F S)
40 Directory of food and nutrition institutions in the Near East, 1987 (E)
41 Residues of some veterinary drugs in animals and foods, 1988 (E)
41/2 Residues of some veterinary drugs in animals and foods. Thirty-fourth meeting of the joint FAO/WHO Expert Committee on Food Additives, 1990 (E)
41/3 Residues of some veterinary drugs in animals and foods. Thirty-sixth meeting of the joint FAO/WHO Expert Committee on Food Additives, 1991 (E)
41/4 Residues of some veterinary drugs in animals and foods. Thirty-eighth meeting of the joint FAO/WHO Expert Committee on Food Additives, 1991 (E)
41/5 Residues of some veterinary drugs in animals and foods, 1993 (E)
42 Traditional food plants, 1988 (E)
42/1 Edible plants of Uganda. The value of wild and cultivated plants as food, 1989 (E)

43	Guidelines for agricultural training curricula in Arab countries, 1988 (Ar)
44	Review of food consumption surveys 1988, 1988 (E)
45	Exposure of infants and children to lead, 1989 (E)
46	Street foods, 1990 (E/F/S)
47/1	Utilization of tropical foods: cereals, 1989 (E F S)
47/2	Utilization of tropical foods: roots and tubers, 1989 (E F S)
47/3	Utilization of tropical foods: trees, 1989 (E F S)
47/4	Utilization of tropical foods: tropical beans, 1989 (E F S)
47/5	Utilization of tropical foods: tropical oil seeds, 1989 (E F S)
47/6	Utilization of tropical foods: sugars, spices and stimulants, 1989 (E F S)
47/7	Utilization of tropical foods: fruits and leaves, 1990 (E F S)
47/8	Utilization of tropical foods: animal products, 1990 (E F S)
48	Residues of some veterinary drugs in animals and foods, 1990 (E)
49	JECFA specifications for identity and purity of certain food additives, 1990 (E)
50	Traditional foods in the Near East, 1991 (E)
51	Protein quality evaluation. Report of the joint FAO/WHO Expert Consultation, 1991 (E)
52	Compendium of food additive specifications - Addendum 1, 1992 (E)
53	Meat and meat products in human nutrition in developing countries, 1992 (E)

Availability: January 1993

Ar	–	Arabic	Multil –	Multilingual
C	–	Chinese	*	Out of print
E	–	English	**	In preparation
F	–	French		
P	–	Portuguese		
S	–	Spanish		

The FAO Technical Papers are available through the authorized FAO Sales Agents or directly from Distribution and Sales Section, FAO, Viale delle Terme di Caracalla, 00100 Rome, Italy.